The Blue Connection

Longevity, Well-Being, and the Power of Water

Peter T Fayette

© Copyright 2024 - All rights reserved.

The content contained within this book may not be reproduced, duplicated or transmitted without direct written permission from the author or the publisher.

Under no circumstances will any blame or legal responsibility be held against the publisher, or author, for any damages, reparation, or monetary loss due to the information contained within this book, either directly or indirectly.

Legal Notice:

This book is copyright protected. It is only for personal use. You cannot amend, distribute, sell, use, quote or paraphrase any part, or the content within this book, without the consent of the author or publisher.

Disclaimer Notice:

Please note the information contained within this document is for educational and entertainment purposes only. All effort has been executed to present accurate, up to date, reliable, complete information. No warranties of any kind are declared or implied. Readers acknowledge that the author is not engaged in the rendering of legal, financial, medical or professional advice. The content within this book has been derived from various sources. Please consult a licensed professional before attempting any techniques outlined in this book.

By reading this document, the reader agrees that under no circumstances is the author responsible for any losses, direct or indirect, that are incurred as a result of the use of the information contained within this document, including, but not limited to, errors, omissions, or inaccuracies.

Table of Contents

FOREWORD 1

INTRODUCTION 3

FIVE BLUE ZONE AREAS 3
A HOLISTIC APPROACH TO LIFE 4
LET'S EXPLORE THE BLUE CONNECTION TOGETHER! 5

CHAPTER 1: INTRODUCTION TO THE BLUE ZONES AND BLUE MIND CONCEPTS 7

OVERVIEW OF BLUE ZONES 8
Okinawa, Japan 8
Sardinia, Italy 11
Nicoya, Costa Rica 15
Ikaria, Greece 18
Loma Linda, California 22
THE BLUE CONNECTION 25
The Benefit of Being Near Water 26
The Blue Zone Lifestyle 28
BRINGING IT ALL TOGETHER 31

CHAPTER 2: THE SCIENCE OF LONGEVITY AND HAPPINESS ... 33

BIOLOGICAL UNDERPINNINGS OF LONGEVITY 33
Regular Physical Activity Contributes to Longevity 34
A Healthy Diet Contributes to a Long and Healthy Life ... 35
Creating Social Connections Leads to Long and Happy Life 38
Low-Stress Levels Promote Longer Lifespans 41
THE ROLE OF GOOD GENES 44
Sirtuin Genes 44
Cholesterol Metabolism 45
Telomeres 45

Epigenetics 45

COMBINED EFFECTS OF VARIOUS FACTORS IMPROVE QUALITY OF LIFE
.... 46

Intergenerational Bonds and Nutrient-Rich Diets 46

Mediterranean Diet, Active Lifestyle, and Relaxation 46

Positive Outlook, Social Bonds, and a Nutrient-Rich Diet
.... 47

Active Lifestyles, Nutrient-Rich Diets, and Strong Social
Bonds 47

Faith, Vegetarianism, and Community Cohesion for
Longevity 48

INTEGRATING SCIENCE AND LIFESTYLE 48

CONCLUDING THOUGHTS 49

**CHAPTER 3: SUBCONSCIOUS AWARENESS OF WATER
PROXIMITY 51**

SENSORY INPUT BEYOND SIGHT 51

We Can Smell Water 52

We Can Hear Water Sources 53

We Can Feel Nearby Water 55

MY PERSONAL CONNECTION TO WATER 56

EVOLUTIONARY ADAPTATION AND PHYSIOLOGICAL CHANGES 56

Relaxing Effects of Water 57

We Seek Water for Relief 57

Water Therapies 58

FINAL INSIGHTS 60

**CHAPTER 4: COMMUNITY AND CONNECTION IN BLUE SPACES
.... 63**

SOCIAL FABRIC OF BLUE ZONES 63

Reduces Stress Levels and Increases Satisfaction 64

Contributes to Longevity and Mental Health 64

Promotes Healthier Lifestyles 65

CREATING BLUE ZONE COMMUNITIES IN BLUE MIND ENVIRONMENTS
.... 65

Casual Meet-Ups Near Water 66

Water-Focused Groups or Clubs 67

Educational Workshops 70

Kids' Programs 72

Consider Inclusivity 73

WATER HAS SHAPED MY LIFE, MY JOURNEY 75

FINAL THOUGHTS 76

CHAPTER 5: PURPOSE AND BLUE MINDFUL LIVING 77

PURPOSE IN BLUE ZONES 77

The Science Behind Purpose 78

Having a Purpose Encourages Positive Behaviors 78

Defining Your Purpose Through Mindfulness 79

FINDING PURPOSE THROUGH WATER 81

Have a Specific Intention in Mind 81

Engage in Purposeful Tasks 83

Choose Meaningful Water Activities 84

Incorporate Water Rituals 85

Encourage Children to Join Water-Related Activities 87

MY FIRST EXPERIENCE WITH WATER 88

FINAL THOUGHTS 89

CHAPTER 6: MOVEMENT AND WATER-INSPIRED ACTIVITIES 91

MOVEMENT IN BLUE ZONES: NATURAL, LOW-INTENSITY DAILY
PHYSICAL ACTIVITIES 91

Walking 92

Gardening 93

Manual Tasks 95

Mental Benefits of Physical Activities 97

BENEFITS OF WATER-BASED MOVEMENT: PHYSICAL AND MENTAL
HEALTH BENEFITS OF AQUATIC EXERCISES 99

*Swimming and Aqua Aerobics Are Great Forms of
Exercise* 99

Buoyancy Prevents Strain on the Body 101

Mental Health Benefits 101

Integrate Physical Activities in Your Daily Routines 101

THE DAY MY MIND TURNED BLUE 102

FINAL THOUGHTS 102

CHAPTER 7: DIET, HYDRATION, AND THE HEALING POWER OF WATER 105

BLUE ZONES DIET PRINCIPLES AND AQUATIC FOODS FOR LONGEVITY
.... 105
   Plant-Based Nutrition 106
   Vegetables and Fruits 107
   No Processed Foods 108
   Occasional Meat 110
   Seafood and Water-Sourced Foods 111
WATER'S ROLE IN DIET AND PRACTICAL STEPS FOR HYDRATION 112
   Drink Only Quality Water Sources 112
   Avoid Sugary Drinks 113
   Eating Water-Rich Foods 114
SUMMARY AND REFLECTIONS 116

CHAPTER 8: REST, RELAXATION, AND BLUE MINDFULNESS 117

REST AND RELAXATION IN BLUE ZONES 117
   Naps Reset the Body 118
   A Relaxing Lifestyle 118
   Daily Downtime 119
   Embracing Leisure 119
   Mindful Moments 120
INCORPORATING BLUE MIND PRACTICES INTO DAILY LIFE 120
   Take Calming Baths 120
   Listen to Water 122
   Visit Local Bodies of Water 123
CONCLUDING THOUGHTS 123

CHAPTER 9: CREATING YOUR PERSONAL BLUE ZONE WITH BLUE MIND PRINCIPLES 125

DESIGNING YOUR ENVIRONMENT 125
   Choose Calming Colors 126
   Adding Natural Elements 127
   Having Ample Lighting 128
   Comfortable Furniture Arrangement 130
FINAL INSIGHTS 131

CHAPTER 10: CHALLENGES AND SOLUTIONS IN MODERN LIFE
.... 133

OBSTACLES TO BLUE ZONE AND BLUE MIND LIVING 133
OVERCOMING BARRIERS USING TECHNOLOGY AND WATER THERAPY
.... 134
Virtual Water Experience 135
Water Visualization 136
Using Technology and Apps 137
Water Therapy 139
FINAL THOUGHTS 141

CHAPTER 11: THE FUTURE OF BLUE LIVING 143

MY FAMILY'S LEGACY ON LAKE CHAMPLAIN 143
POTENTIAL FOR URBAN BLUE ZONES 144
Adding Natural Water Sources to Cityscapes 144
Green Infrastructure 146
Sustainable Architectural Practices 148
BLUE MIND AND PUBLIC HEALTH ADVOCACY 150
Create Equitable Access 150
Supporting Conservation Efforts 152
Community Participation 153
Enhancing Mental and Physical Health 155
MEDICAL BREAKTHROUGHS 156
Rapamycin Overview 156
Key Findings on Rapamycin's Impact on Longevity 157
Side Effects and Future Directions 157
FINAL THOUGHTS 158
BRINGING IT ALL TOGETHER 158

CONCLUSION 161

LET'S CREATE BLUE ZONES IN OUR COMMUNITIES 161
IMPROVE HEALTH AND WELLNESS WITH BLUE MIND WISDOM 162
PROMOTE ACCESS TO CLEAN DRINKING WATER 163
SUPPORT INITIATIVES TO PROTECT BODIES OF WATER 163
CONSIDERING MEDICAL BREAKTHROUGHS 164
CREATING SPACES AND LIFESTYLES THAT HONOR THE IMPORTANCE OF
WATER 165

The Power of Water Is Within Us...........................166

REFERENCES 167

To Wallace 'J' Nichols, marine biologist, author, and the visionary behind the Blue Mind movement.

Your work has shown us how deeply connected we are to water, reminding us of the peace, joy, and health it brings to our lives. This book is a tribute to your passion and dedication, blending the wisdom of Blue Zones with the healing power of Blue Mind to guide us toward a healthier, more connected life. You helped me understand something I could never quite put into words about my own love of water.

Thank you for showing us the calming, healing blue that surrounds us all. You are missed, my friend.

Foreword

When I first came across the concept of Blue Zones—those remarkable pockets of the world where people live significantly longer and healthier lives—I was intrigued. However, as I researched, one detail stood out to me: four of the five Blue Zones are located near bodies of water, with three being islands.

Yet, in all the discussions about diet, community, and lifestyle, water was not identified as a key factor contributing to longevity.

Having been a member of the *Blue Mind Book Club* for the past five years, I was already familiar with the transformative impact of water on the human mind and body. Through my ongoing dialogue with J. Nichols, the author of *Blue Mind*, I became increasingly convinced that water—whether through proximity or interaction—plays a crucial role in enhancing mental clarity, emotional well-being, and overall life satisfaction, fostering a deeper connection between humans and nature.

I even attempted to bring the authors of the Blue Zones research to the Blue Mind table, hoping we could explore this idea further. Their response, however, was that while they acknowledged the stress-reducing properties of water, they were not interested in pursuing a joint research project on the subject. That response left me unsatisfied.

I felt there was so much more to uncover.

So, I decided to pursue this exploration myself, and this book is the result of that journey.

In *The Blue Connection*, I invite you to discover how our relationship with water could be the missing link in our understanding of longevity and well-being. What follows is my attempt to bring together the science, stories, and personal insights that highlight the power of water in shaping our lives for the better.

Introduction

In today's fast-paced and often stressed-out world, the search for a longer, healthier, and more fulfilling life has led many to explore unique lifestyles and habits that promote well-being.

Among these are the fascinating concepts of Blue Zones and Blue Mind, two distinct yet intriguingly connected ways of living that offer profound insights into achieving longevity and enhancing mental and physical health.

Imagine a place where people live significantly longer than average, enjoying vitality and joy well into their 90s or even over 100 years old. These remarkable regions of the world are known as Blue Zones.

Five Blue Zone Areas

Researchers have identified five such areas: Okinawa in Japan, Sardinia in Italy, Ikaria in Greece, Loma Linda in California, and the Nicoya Peninsula in Costa Rica. What sets these regions apart are the common lifestyle characteristics shared by their inhabitants—factors that contribute to their extraordinary longevity and quality of life:

- diet

- community

- movement

- sense of purpose

- relaxation and stress reduction

As we shift our focus from land to water, the concept of Blue Mind introduces us to the incredible benefits of being near or in aquatic environments. Water has a unique ability to soothe and invigorate simultaneously, offering a powerful antidote to the pressures of modern life.

Being near water can lead to a state of 'Blue Mind,' characterized by feelings of calm, peace, unity, and a sense of general happiness with life in the moment.

A Holistic Approach to Life

Combining the principles of Blue Zones and Blue Mind creates a holistic approach to well-being that is both compelling and practical. The synergy between these concepts lies in their mutual reinforcement of healthful practices that address both body and mind.

By integrating aspects of Blue Zones with the tranquility and rejuvenation offered by Blue Mind, one can cultivate a balanced, fulfilling lifestyle that promotes longevity and wellness.

Let's Explore the Blue Connection Together!

This book explores how adopting a blend of Blue Zones and Blue Mind recommendations can transform your life. We will delve into real-life examples, provide actionable advice, and share inspiring stories of communities and individuals who embody these principles.

You'll discover that this integrative approach doesn't require drastic changes but encourages mindful adjustments that align with your existing lifestyle.

By embracing the wisdom of Blue Zones and the serenity of Blue Mind, this book guides you towards a vibrant, healthier, and more joyful existence.

We invite you to explore these concepts deeply, implement these teachings, and witness firsthand the transformative power of living a life inspired by the world's healthiest and happiest places! Let's go!

Chapter 1:

Introduction to the Blue Zones and Blue Mind Concepts

Blue Zones, regions identified for their high concentration of centenarians, offer valuable insights into diet, community engagement, and physical activity that promote long, healthy lives.

Let's focus on the core attributes of Blue Zones and unravel the essence of the Blue Mind concept, which highlights the mental and emotional benefits of being near water. Explore how the tranquil presence of water can lower stress levels, enhance creativity, and foster a sense of peace.

Overview of Blue Zones

Recognized for their remarkable longevity and the well-being of their inhabitants, these regions provide a wealth of insights into living a long and healthy life.

Okinawa, Japan

Okinawa, Japan, is perhaps the most famous of the Blue Zones, widely recognized for the extraordinary longevity and vitality of its residents. People in Okinawa often live well into their 90s and beyond, with many remaining active, mentally sharp, and socially engaged throughout their later years. Their exceptional health outcomes reveal key lifestyle and cultural practices that contribute to their remarkable longevity.

One of the central concepts of the Okinawan way of life is "Ikigai," which translates to "reason for being" or "a reason to wake up in the morning." This deep sense of purpose gives Okinawans a strong drive to live meaningfully and stay connected with their community, family, and activities that bring them joy. Research suggests that this sense of purpose boosts mental well-being, reduces stress, lowers the risk of heart disease, and helps maintain mental acuity as they age (Bishop, 2023).

Dietary Habits

Dietary habits in Okinawa are another cornerstone of their longevity. Their traditional diet is heavily plant-based, consisting primarily of:

- Vegetables like leafy greens, seaweed, and cruciferous vegetables.

- Tofu and other soy-based products, which are rich in plant protein and contain isoflavones that support cardiovascular health and hormone balance.

- Sweet potatoes, a dietary staple, are rich in fiber, antioxidants, and complex carbohydrates that provide sustained energy and support digestive health.

- Fish is a primary source of protein and omega-3 fatty acids, known for their anti-inflammatory properties and role in maintaining heart and brain health.

Notably, Okinawans consume very little meat and dairy products, which are often linked to higher risks of chronic diseases in Western diets. Instead, their emphasis on nutrient-dense, low-calorie foods promotes longevity while minimizing the risk of obesity, diabetes, and cardiovascular diseases.

Moderation

Moderation is also key in Okinawan eating habits, with a cultural practice known as "Hara Hachi Bu," meaning, "eat until you are 80% full." This mindful approach to eating helps prevent overeating and supports digestive efficiency, contributing to weight management and metabolic health. Combined with their active lifestyle, Okinawans enjoy sustained energy levels and metabolic efficiency throughout their lives.

Physical Activity

Physical activity is seamlessly woven into the Okinawan way of life. Rather than participating in structured exercise routines, daily movement is natural and frequent. Activities such as walking, gardening, and maintaining household tasks keep them physically fit without the need for intense workouts. This type of movement, which involves endurance, strength, and flexibility, promotes cardiovascular health, muscle tone, and overall mobility, allowing the elderly to remain independent and active.

Social Connections

Strong social connections are vital to Okinawan health. The concept of "Moai," or close-knit social groups, fosters a strong sense of community and provides emotional support throughout life's challenges. These social bonds are believed to reduce stress, increase happiness, and even extend life expectancy by promoting a sense of belonging and security.

Cultural Practices

Cultural practices such as respect for elders, daily mindfulness, and the preservation of traditional customs further enhance Okinawan longevity by promoting mental well-being and reinforcing a sense of identity. Combined with Okinawa's natural environment, where residents are often surrounded by tranquil landscapes and the calming presence of the sea, their lifestyle creates a harmonious balance between mind, body, and spirit.

Sardinia, Italy

Sardinia, a rugged island off the coast of Italy, is another renowned Blue Zone where inhabitants enjoy some of the highest concentrations of male centenarians in the world. Sardinians maintain a rich cultural heritage that prioritizes traditional living, with a lifestyle rooted in agriculture, family, and community. Their unique combination of diet, physical activity, and strong social bonds contributes significantly to their impressive longevity and quality of life.

Physical Activity

Physical activity is naturally integrated into Sardinian life, much like in other Blue Zones. Many Sardinians, particularly the men, are involved in farming and raising livestock, tasks that keep them physically active well into their old age. This daily activity strengthens their bodies and maintains cardiovascular health, muscle tone, and bone density. The terrain of Sardinia, marked by steep hills and valleys, requires regular walking and climbing, further adding to their endurance and physical resilience.

Diet

The Sardinian diet plays a role in their longevity. It is simple but nutrient-rich, relying on locally sourced, natural foods. Their traditional meals include:

- Whole grains such as barley and wheat, which are often used in breads and pastas. These grains are packed with fiber, helping regulate blood sugar levels and supporting digestive health.

- Beans such as fava beans and chickpeas are staples in Sardinian cuisine, providing an affordable and nutritious source of plant-based protein, fiber, and essential vitamins. Beans have been linked to reduced heart disease and other chronic conditions (Vieira, 2023).

- Garden vegetables including tomatoes, zucchini, and potatoes are grown locally and consumed in abundance. These vegetables supply essential vitamins, minerals, and antioxidants that support overall health and reduce inflammation.

- Pecorino cheese, made from the milk of grass-fed sheep, is a unique feature of the Sardinian diet. This cheese is rich in omega-3 fatty acids, which have anti-inflammatory properties and contribute to cardiovascular health. Pecorino is consumed in moderation, often paired with other nutrient-dense foods, ensuring the diet remains balanced and varied.

Another notable part of the Sardinian lifestyle is wine consumption, particularly Cannonau wine. This red wine is known for its high levels of antioxidants, specifically resveratrol and polyphenols, which have been linked to heart health and longevity. Wine in Sardinia is consumed in moderation, typically with meals, and always in a social setting. Sharing wine during family gatherings or community events reinforces social bonds and provides a sense of togetherness, both of which are critical to emotional well-being.

Social Connections

Social cohesion is another factor in the Sardinian way of life. Family is central to their culture, and elderly family members are not only cared for but revered. Grandparents play an active role in the upbringing of their grandchildren, fostering a strong sense of intergenerational connection and mutual support. This respect for elders and close-knit family structures helps reduce loneliness and stress, both of which are known to influence overall health.

Community

Aside from family, community involvement is important to Sardinian life. Locals engage in frequent social interactions with neighbors and friends, whether through communal meals, religious gatherings, or festivals. This sense of belonging and shared purpose is linked to lower stress levels, improved mental health, and an increased sense of happiness.

Slow-Paced Life

Sardinians also benefit from a slow pace of life that emphasizes relaxation and enjoying the moment. Unlike fast-paced modern societies, Sardinians prioritize downtime, whether it's enjoying a long meal, taking a midday rest, or spending time in nature. This focus on relaxation helps mitigate the harmful effects of chronic stress, contributing to a longer healthier life.

Spirituality

Spirituality and tradition also play a significant role in Sardinian life. Many Sardinians attend church regularly, and religious festivals are central to their community's social fabric. This deep sense of spirituality offers psychological comfort, fostering hope, gratitude, and a positive outlook in life.

Nicoya, Costa Rica

Nicoya, a peninsula in northwestern Costa Rica, is another fascinating Blue Zone where residents experience remarkably long and healthy lives. The Nicoyan people attribute their exceptional longevity to a combination of lifestyle factors deeply rooted in their cultural and natural environment.

Key elements of their life include strong family ties, a nutrient-rich diet, regular physical activity, and a connection to nature, all of which contribute to their physical, mental, and emotional well-being.

One of the most significant aspects of life in Nicoya is its strong sense of family and community. Family is the cornerstone of Nicoyan culture, and elders are revered and cared for within the family unit. This intergenerational support provides a sense of purpose and belonging for older adults, reducing feelings of loneliness and stress. The community as a whole shares a close bond, with frequent social gatherings and mutual assistance, which reinforces emotional security and promotes mental health.

Diet

The Nicoyan diet is another key contributor to their longevity. It consists of traditional, whole foods that are nutrient-dense and minimally processed. Some of the staples include:

- Beans, especially black beans, are consumed daily and provide a rich source of plant-based protein, fiber, and essential vitamins. This reduces the risk of heart disease and helps maintain steady energy levels.

- Corn is another dietary staple, often eaten in the form of tortillas or tamales. Corn provides complex carbohydrates and fiber, supporting digestion and blood sugar control.

- Squash and other locally grown vegetables such as yucca and plantains, contribute to a diet rich in vitamins, minerals, and antioxidants. These vegetables provide important nutrients such as beta-carotene and potassium, which support heart health and reduce inflammation.

- Tropical fruits like papayas, oranges, and bananas are abundant in the region and consumed regularly. These fruits are packed with antioxidants, vitamins, and natural sugars that provide energy and protect against disease.

One unique aspect of Nicoyan health is their water supply, which is high in calcium and magnesium. These minerals are essential for bone health and cardiovascular function, helping to reduce the risk of osteoporosis and heart disease, both are critical in aging populations.

Physical Activity

Physical activity is seamlessly integrated into daily life in Nicoya. Many Nicoyans are involved in agricultural work, which requires regular movement, strength, and endurance. Tasks such as planting, harvesting, and tending to livestock keep them physically active well into old age. In addition, walking is a primary mode of transportation, with many residents walking long distances as part of their daily routines. This promotes cardiovascular health, builds muscle, and maintains flexibility without the need for structured workouts.

A Positive Outlook

Another factor contributing to Nicoyan's longevity is their positive outlook in life. Nicoyans often express a sense of "Plan de Vida," which is similar to Okinawa's Ikigai, referring to their sense of purpose in life. Whether it's through maintaining their farms, caring for grandchildren, or participating in community events, having a clear sense of purpose gives Nicoyans a reason to stay active and engaged throughout their lives.

Stress Reducing Lifestyle

Nicoyans have a relaxed pace of life, combined with a natural environment rich in green landscapes and proximity to the ocean. These help lower stress levels and promote emotional well-being. Daily practices such as prayer, mindfulness, and spending time with family contribute to their ability to manage stress more effectively.

Spirituality

Many residents practice religion regularly. This deep connection to faith offers comfort, resilience, and emotional stability, especially in challenging times. It also fosters a strong sense of community, with religious gatherings serving as an opportunity for socialization and mutual support.

Ikaria, Greece

Known as "The island where people forget to die," Ikaria is a Greek island in the Aegean Sea that boasts one of the highest percentages of centenarians in the world. This region boasts a remarkably low rate of dementia and other chronic diseases (Buettner, 2012). The people of Ikaria have remarkable longevity and health because of a harmonious blend of diet, lifestyle, and social structure, all rooted in traditional practices that have been passed down for generations.

Diet

The Ikarian diet is central to their health and longevity. It follows a Mediterranean pattern, which is rich in plant-based foods, and low in processed ingredients. Key elements of the Ikarian diet include:

- Legumes such as chickpeas, lentils, and beans are consumed frequently, providing a significant source of plant-based protein, fiber, and essential nutrients such as magnesium and potassium. These legumes are associated with reduced risks of heart disease and diabetes, key factors in healthy aging.

- Wild greens such as dandelions and purslane are gathered locally and are staples in Ikarian meals. These are incredibly nutrient-dense, offering high levels of antioxidants, vitamins, and anti-inflammatory properties. They contribute to overall health by supporting immune function and reducing oxidative stress.

- Goat's milk is commonly consumed and offers an excellent source of calcium, vitamin D, and probiotics, all of which support bone health and gut function. Goat's milk is easier to digest than cow's milk and has anti-inflammatory properties, which may explain why Ikarian elders maintain strong bones and muscle mass into old age.

- Fresh fish is another important part of the Ikarian diet, providing a rich source of omega-3 fatty acids that support heart health, reduce inflammation, and contribute to cognitive function. Fish, such as sardines and mackerel are typically grilled or prepared simply, preserving their nutrient content.

- Olive oil is a staple in Ikarian cooking, used generously in salads, stews, and other dishes. Olive oil is rich in heart-healthy monosaturated fats and antioxidants, particularly oleic acid, which has been linked to reduced inflammation and protection against heart disease. Its regular use may be one of the reasons Ikarians enjoy such low rates of cardiovascular issues.

Siesta

Beyond diet, the slow-paced, stress-free lifestyle of Ikaria is crucial to their longevity. The island's inhabitants prioritize relaxation and mindfulness, often taking afternoon naps or "siesta." This daily rest lowers stress levels, improves mood, and reduces the risk of heart-related conditions by lowering blood pressure. Unlike fast-paced urban environments, Ikaria promotes life in balance, where people focus on enjoying the present rather than rushing through their days.

Physical Activity

Rather than structured exercise routines, Ikarians stay active through gardening, walking, and maintaining their homes. The island's hilly terrain encourages natural movement, as residents must often walk long distances on steep paths to reach neighbors or shops. This type of low-intensity, consistent movement strengthens muscles, promotes cardiovascular health, and supports joint flexibility; allowing Ikarians to remain physically capable even in their later years.

Social Connections

The island has a rich tradition of communal gatherings, where residents come together for festivals, meals, and religious events. These frequent social interactions foster a sense of belonging and emotional support, which has been shown to reduce stress and improve mental health.

The strong sense of community also provides a safety net for elders, who are never left to feel isolated and alone. The concept of "filoxenia" or hospitality is deeply ingrained in Ikarian culture, with neighbors and friends frequently stopping by each other's homes, offering companionship and care.

Spirituality

Many of the island's residents attend church regularly and participate in religious festivals. This connection to faith provides a sense of purpose and a calming influence on mental and emotional well-being. The regular practice of mindfulness, prayer, and gratitude helps Ikarians cope with life's challenges, reducing the impact of stress and enhancing their overall outlook on life.

Connection to Nature

Surrounded by lush landscapes and the tranquil Aegean Sea, the island's natural beauty offers a sense of peace and relaxation. Ikarians spend much of their time outdoors, whether tending to gardens or socializing in village squares, further supporting their mental and physical health.

Loma Linda, California

Loma Linda, California, is unique among the Blue Zones because it is home to a concentrated community of Seventh-day Adventists. It is also the only Blue Zone that is not located near any body of water. Despite this, the residents here have successfully cultivated habits that lead to long and healthy lives, largely rooted in their faith-based principles.

Diet

The Seventh-day Adventist lifestyle centers on the concept of holistic health, which integrates spiritual, physical, and mental well-being. A major aspect of this lifestyle is the biblical diet, which emphasizes plant-based eating and the avoidance of substances such as alcohol, tobacco, and caffeinated beverages. This dietary approach is considered essential to maintaining health and preventing disease.

Key elements of the Adventist diet include:

- Nuts and seeds are consumed regularly, providing a rich source of healthy fats, fiber, and protein. These foods are associated with reduced inflammation, improved heart health, and lower cholesterol levels, all of which contribute to the Adventists' impressive longevity.

- Fruits and vegetables are abundant providing essential vitamins, minerals, and antioxidants that support overall health and protect against chronic disease. Their emphasis on colorful, seasonal produce ensures they receive a wide range of nutrients.

- Whole grains such as oats, brown rice, and barley are staple foods, offering complex carbohydrates and fiber that support digestive health and stabilize blood sugar levels. These provide long-lasting energy, reducing the need for processed or sugary foods.

- Legumes including beans, lentils, and peas are regularly incorporated into meals, offering plant-based protein and essential nutrients such as iron and magnesium. These legumes contribute to heart health and help maintain muscle mass, particularly as individuals age.

No Alcohol and Tobacco

This practice protects against diseases such as cancer and liver disease and promotes a culture of self-discipline and health consciousness. By avoiding these harmful substances, Adventists significantly lower their risk for chronic illnesses, which is reflected in their extended lifespans.

Physical Activity

Regular exercise is encouraged but is often integrated into daily routines rather than through structured workouts. Many Adventists enjoy hiking, walking, and gardening, activities that promote cardiovascular health and maintain muscle and joint flexibility. The surrounding natural environment, with its hiking trails and outdoor spaces, encourages residents to stay active and connected to nature.

Community Bond

The church plays a central role in fostering these connections, providing a space for fellowship and mutual support. Members of the Loma Linda community come together for social events, religious services, and volunteer activities, all of which strengthen their bonds and offer emotional support. This sense of belonging and purpose significantly contributes to mental and emotional well-being, helping to reduce stress and promote a positive outlook on life.

Sabbath

One of the most important rituals in the Adventist community is the weekly observance of the Sabbath. Every week, from sunset on Friday to sunset on Saturday, Adventists observe a day of rest known as the Shabbat.

During this time, work is set aside in favor of spiritual reflection, prayer, and spending time with family and friends. This restorative break from daily stress provides a crucial opportunity for mental and physical recuperation, promoting longevity by reducing stress.

Spiritual Health

Adventists also prioritize spiritual health as an essential part of their overall well-being. Their faith emphasizes living with a sense of purpose and a commitment to caring for the body as a temple. This spiritual outlook encourages Adventists to adopt healthy habits, avoid harmful substances, and engage in activities that promote long-term well-being. The integration of faith and health gives them a strong foundation for living fulfilling purpose-driven lives.

The Blue Connection

The Blue Connection merges the profound principles of Blue Zones and the Blue Mind, offering a holistic path to longevity and emotional balance. Blue Zones—regions of the world where people live longer and healthier lives—reveal the significance of lifestyle factors such as diet, movement, social connection, and a sense of purpose. Blue Zones embody the idea that health isn't just about avoiding disease but about embracing life fully, with community and routine playing a central role.

Meanwhile, Blue Mind focuses on the mental and emotional health benefits derived from water. Whether it's a vast ocean or a calm river, water has a unique ability to soothe the mind, reduce stress, and enhance creativity. Studies have shown that proximity to water encourages mindfulness, lowers cortisol levels, and nurtures emotional well-being (Zhang, 2021).

By integrating the lessons of physical longevity from Blue Zones with the mental tranquility of Blue Mind, we create a well-rounded approach to wellness. This synthesis doesn't just target physical vitality or mental clarity in isolation but brings them together in a way that acknowledges how deeply interconnected our bodies and minds truly are. The result is a comprehensive strategy for living a longer, more fulfilled and peaceful life where healthy habits and a connection to nature form the foundation of lasting well-being.

The Benefit of Being Near Water

The Blue Mind concept emphasizes the profound psychological and physiological benefits of proximity to water. Research has shown that being near bodies of water can reduce stress, enhance creativity, and promote an overall sense of calmness (Zhang, et al., 2021).

Whether it's the gentle sound of waves, the sight of a flowing river, or the sensation of floating in a pool, water has the power to trigger positive emotional responses that engage the body's natural relaxation processes. These responses are linked to lower cortisol levels, reduced tension, and an improved mood.

- **Reduced stress levels:** The soothing presence of water helps activate the parasympathetic nervous system, reducing cortisol production and alleviating feelings of stress.

- **Enhanced creativity:** Being near water has been shown to boost creative thinking and problem-solving abilities by promoting mental clarity and relaxation.

- **Improved focus and concentration:** Water environments encourage mindfulness and a deeper state of focus, helping to clear the mental clutter that can inhibit productivity.

- **Lowered blood pressure and heart rate:** The calming sounds and visuals of water can help reduce blood pressure and slow the heart rate, contributing to overall cardiovascular health.

- **Boosted mood and emotional well-being:** Water environments stimulate positive emotional responses, including feelings of happiness, contentment, and tranquility, while reducing anxiety and depression symptoms.

- **Enhanced sleep quality:** Exposure to water can promote better sleep patterns by inducing a calm, relaxed state that is conducive to deeper and more restorative rest.

By spending time near water, you can tap into these amazing benefits, enhancing your mental and physical well-being in a natural and holistic way.

The Blue Zone Lifestyle

The people who live in Blue Zones, such as Okinawa in Japan or Ikaria in Greece, have been observed to live longer and healthier lives. Their lifestyles are rooted in simple, yet profound habits that prioritize physical, social, and emotional health. These populations follow practices that naturally foster well-being and significantly reduce the risk of chronic diseases.

Key factors of the Blue Zone lifestyle include:

- **Plant-based diets, rich in nutrients:** Blue Zone inhabitants consume mostly whole foods, including vegetables, fruits, legumes, and grains, with limited amounts of meat. This nutrient-dense, anti-inflammatory diet is critical to long-term health.

- **Regular, low-intensity physical activity:** Instead of structured exercise routines, daily movement is part of life in Blue Zones. Whether it's gardening, walking, or manual tasks, physical activity is naturally embedded in their routines, promoting cardiovascular health and muscular endurance.

- **Strong social connections:** A sense of belonging and community is central to Blue Zone cultures. Their close-knit communities foster emotional support, which has been linked to lower stress levels and better mental health outcomes.

- **Sense of purpose ("Ikigai" or "Plan de Vida"):** People in Blue Zones have a clearly defined sense of purpose, which gives them motivation to live longer and more meaningful lives. This sense of purpose is seen as a critical factor in maintaining mental resilience and vitality.

- **Moderate alcohol consumption:** In several Blue Zones, moderate consumption of wine, particularly during meals is common. This social, mindful approach to alcohol, especially red wine rich in antioxidants, contributes to heart health when consumed responsibly.

- **Stress reduction rituals:** Blue Zone inhabitants incorporate daily practices to reduce stress, such as napping, prayer, meditation, or enjoying social time with loved ones. These routines help lower inflammation and improve overall health.

- **Respect for elders:** Elders are highly valued in Blue Zone communities, playing active roles in both family and society. This respect and intergenerational connection offer a sense of continuity and purpose, benefiting both younger and older generations.

- **Proximity to nature:** Blue Zones tend to be located in regions with abundant natural beauty, from mountains to seas. Regular exposure to nature is linked to improved mental health, enhanced mood, and physical activity.

When the lifestyle principles of Blue Zones are combined with the water-related relaxation benefits of the Blue Mind, a unique synergy happens. Together, they offer a comprehensive, balanced approach to physical health, mental well-being, and emotional fulfillment, creating a blueprint for long, vibrant lives.

Bringing It All Together

Blue Zones and Blue Mind principles are fascinating. By examining these unique regions, we've identified key lifestyle habits that contribute to holistic health.

The emphasis on plant-based diets, strong community ties, and natural physical activity in Blue Zones, combined with the stress-reducing, mood-enhancing effects of proximity to water, offers a comprehensive approach to enhancing physical and mental well-being.

Embracing the synergy between the Blue Zones' enduring lifestyles and the restorative power of Blue Mind can lead to a more balanced and fulfilling life.

Chapter 2:

The Science of Longevity and Happiness

From diet and physical activity to social connections and stress management, each factor plays a crucial role in fostering a life full of vitality and contentment in Blue Zones. By understanding these elements, you can integrate science-backed practices into your own life, paving the way to a happier and longer life.

Biological Underpinnings of Longevity

Longevity is influenced by a blend of lifestyle habits, social connections, stress management, and genetic factors. When studying Blue Zones—regions where people live significantly longer lives—these elements are clearly evident.

Regular Physical Activity Contributes to Longevity

In Blue Zones, physical activity is an integral part of everyday life, seamlessly woven into routine tasks rather than through structured workouts at the gym. The concept of "incidental exercise" is common in these regions, where people engage in consistent, low-intensity movement throughout their day. This activity is effortless yet effective, promoting longevity by maintaining the body's health and vitality over time.

Walking

For instance, residents of Blue Zones may walk several miles a day, whether to visit neighbors, fetch groceries, or simply enjoy their surroundings. In places such as Ikaria, the hilly terrain ensures that walking requires more effort, making it a natural form of cardiovascular exercise.

Farming

Similarly, in Sardinia, men and women often engage in farming, tending to livestock, or harvesting crops, all of which involve manual labor and contribute to their physical fitness. These activities provide strength training and flexibility without the need for dedicated gym sessions.

Gardening

Gardening is another common activity across Blue Zones, offering both physical and mental benefits. In Okinawa, many elderly residents maintain personal vegetable gardens, bending, squatting, and digging regularly. These movements help preserve joint flexibility, improve circulation, and reduce the risk of osteoporosis, all while providing fresh produce to support their nutritious diets. Gardening also offers a sense of purpose and connection to nature, contributing to emotional well-being.

Natural Environment

This natural environment is sustainable and achievable across all ages. Unlike high-intensity exercises that can become difficult with age, the daily movements of walking, gardening, or performing household chores are gentle yet effective. This constant, low-intensity activity maintains cardiovascular health, improves muscle strength, and preserves mobility well into old age.

A Healthy Diet Contributes to a Long and Healthy Life

In all Blue Zones, a healthy diet is a cornerstone of longevity, playing a vital role in supporting physical health, preventing chronic diseases, and promoting vitality into old age. The residents of these regions have developed dietary patterns that are rich in natural, whole foods and low in processed or refined ingredients. This focus on nutrient-dense, plant-based diets ensures that their bodies receive the essential nutrients needed to maintain health and prevent diseases.

Plant-Based Eating

Places like Okinawa and Nicoya promote plant-based eating with the majority of their daily calories coming from vegetables, fruits, legumes, and whole grains. These foods are rich in fiber, antioxidants, and anti-inflammatory compounds that protect against diseases such as heart disease, cancer, and diabetes. For example, Okinawans consume large quantities of sweet potatoes that are not only filling but are packed with beta-carotene, a powerful antioxidant that supports eye health and immune function.

Legumes

Beans, lentils, and chickpeas are rich in protein, fiber, and essential nutrients such as iron and magnesium. In Ikaria and Sardinia, legumes are consumed regularly in soups, stews, and salads, providing a plant-based protein source that helps regulate blood sugar levels, reducing the risk of diabetes and other metabolic disorders.

Whole Grains

Whole grains such as oats, barley, and brown rice are vital components of Blue Zone diets. Unlike refined grains, which are stripped of their nutrients, whole grains retain their natural fiber, vitamins, and minerals. This promotes digestive health, stabilizes blood sugar, and provides a steady source of energy throughout the day. In Nicoya, traditional dishes often include corn and squash, which are both nutrient-dense and provide a balanced source of carbohydrates and fiber.

Healthy Fats

Healthy fats are also key to longevity in Blue Zones. In Ikaria and Sardinia, olive oil is used liberally in cooking, offering a rich source of monounsaturated fats and antioxidants, particularly oleic acid, which has been shown to reduce inflammation and support heart health. Healthy fats combined with a diet low in animal products and processed foods, keep cholesterol levels in check and prevent cardiovascular diseases.

Plant-Based Proteins

Protein intake in Blue Zones primarily comes from plant sources although fish is consumed in moderate amounts in coastal areas of Ikaria and Okinawa. Fish such as sardines and mackerel, are rich in omega-3 fatty acids, which support heart health, improve cognitive function, and reduce inflammation. Unlike many Western diets that rely heavily on red meat and processed animal products, Blue Zone diets incorporate lean sources of protein that are less likely to contribute to chronic conditions such as heart disease and cancers.

Local Seasonal Produce

One of the most significant aspects of Blue Zone diets is their reliance on local seasonal produce. Residents eat what is available from their gardens or local farms, ensuring that their food is fresh and free from preservatives or harmful chemicals. This connection to the land not only guarantees the nutritional quality of the food but also fosters a sense of gratitude and appreciation for nature, which in turn contributes to mental and emotional well-being.

Portion Control

In Okinawa, the practice of Hara Hachi Bu, a Confucian teaching that encourages moderation can help prevent overeating and ensure that you consume only the calories needed to maintain energy without overburdening the body. Similarly, in other Blue Zones, meals are typically smaller and spaced throughout the day, preventing the health risks associated with excessive calorie intake.

Creating Social Connections Leads to Long and Happy Life

In Blue Zones, the emphasis on social connections is as vital to longevity as diet and physical activity. People in these regions prioritize familial bonds, friendships, and community integration, creating a strong support network that nurtures both emotional and physical well-being. These relationships are deeply embedded in daily life, contributing to a sense of belonging, purpose, and happiness that is integral to living a long and fulfilling life.

Everyday Interactions

One of the most striking features of Blue Zone communities is how social interactions are naturally woven into everyday activities. Whether it's sharing meals, participating in religious or cultural events, or simply spending time with friends and neighbors, social connections form the foundation of life in these regions. In Okinawa, many residents participate in "Moai" groups, long-term support systems where friends meet regularly to discuss life, share food, and offer help in times of need. This sense of solidarity and mutual support helps reduce stress and fosters a deeper sense of security, knowing they are never alone in facing life's challenges.

Multi-Generational Living

In Sardinia, multi-generational living is common with families often living close to or even in the same households. Grandparents, parents, and children all play a role in each other's lives, creating a strong family unit that provides daily emotional sustenance. These close family ties allow for regular interaction, enabling the elderly to feel valued and connected, while younger generations benefit from the wisdom and experience of their elders. The result is not just a longer lifespan for the elderly but also a richer life experience for all generations.

Friendships

Friendships also play a role in promoting longevity in Blue Zones. In Nicoya, community members often stop by each other's homes for a cup of coffee or a chat, reinforcing the strong social fabric of the region. These casual, frequent interactions help build a sense of belonging and reduce feelings of loneliness and isolation. Having a supportive social network boosts mental resilience and reduces the impact of stress on the body.

Communal Meals

In regions such as Ikaria and Sardinia, meals are rarely eaten alone. Instead, they are occasions to gather with family and friends, reinforcing the bonds that contribute to emotional well-being. In Loma Linda, the Seventh-day Adventist community often shares Sabbath meals, where food and fellowship combine to create a sense of spiritual and emotional rejuvenation. Sharing meals enhances the enjoyment of food and provides an opportunity to connect, laugh, and share experiences, all of which have been shown to reduce cortisol and boost oxytocin, which promotes feelings of trust and emotional warmth.

Group Activities

In Okinawa, elders are often involved in community gardening or Tai Chi classes where they meet with others to engage in physical activity that benefits both the body and mind. In Nicoya, residents are involved in agricultural work and group celebrations, promoting a sense of purpose and teamwork. These group activities maintain physical health but also offer emotional support and a sense of accomplishment, both of which are essential to a happy, long life.

Social Cohesion

In Loma Linda, the Seventh-day Adventist faith encourages community involvement and provides a shared belief system that fosters a sense of purpose and hope. The weekly observance of the Sabbath gives members time for rest, reflection, and connection with others, reinforcing a rhythm of life that prioritizes both physical and mental well-being.

Emotional Sustenance

A supportive network of family and friends prevents stress, which is a significant factor in the development of chronic illnesses including hypertension, heart disease, and depression. The daily acts of love, kindness, and mutual support that are typical in Blue Zones maintain mental health and ensure that individuals feel valued, loved, and part of something greater than themselves.

Low-Stress Levels Promote Longer Lifespans

In the Blue Zones, where the art of living well is honed through generations, low stress levels emerge as a significant contributor to longevity. Unlike the high-stress, fast-paced lifestyles prevalent in many parts of the world, residents in these regions embrace daily routines and practices that foster relaxation and help manage stress effectively. This emphasis on calmness and tranquility reduces the physical and mental burdens that contribute to chronic health issues.

Siestas

In cultures such as those in Nicoya and Sardinia, taking a break during the hottest part of the day is customary. This brief period of rest helps rejuvenate the body and provides an opportunity for the mind to relax and reset. Research indicates that short naps can enhance alertness, improve mood, and even boost cognitive function, allowing you to approach the rest of your day with renewed energy and focus (Lovato, 2010).

Mindfulness Practices

Practices such as prayer and meditation are woven into the fabric of daily life. In Ikaria, many residents engage in spiritual practices that promote reflection and a sense of gratitude. Meditation has been shown to reduce levels of cortisol, the stress hormone while enhancing mental health. These moments of introspection and connection to something greater provide individuals with a sense of purpose and calm.

Moments in Nature

Spending time in nature is another aspect of stress management in Blue Zones. The residents of Okinawa often enjoy outdoor activities whether it's gardening, walking, or sitting near the ocean. These activities lower blood pressure, reduce stress, and enhance feelings of happiness. This connection to the natural environment encourages individuals to slow down, breathe deeply, and appreciate the beauty around them, fostering a sense of peace and well-being.

Social Interactions

The strong social bonds in Blue Zones provide emotional support and a buffer against stress. Spending time with loved ones and friends creates opportunities for laughter, sharing experiences, and discussing challenges, which can all alleviate feelings of anxiety and isolation. The communal nature of life in these regions fosters an atmosphere where individuals feel supported and cared for, allowing them to cope more effectively with stress.

More Personal Time

Residents prioritize relationships, leisure, and personal time over the hustle and bustle that characterizes much of modern living. In Sardinia, the culture places a high value on social gatherings and leisurely meals, where people take their time to enjoy food and company. This unhurried approach allows individuals to savor life's moments and diminishes the pressure to constantly achieve or perform.

Physical Activity

Physical activity in Blue Zones is typically low-intensity and integrated into daily life rather than structured or forced. Whether it's walking to the market, gardening, or engaging in manual labor, these promote physical health while simultaneously providing mental relief. The natural rhythm of these movements allows for a release of endorphins, which are known to enhance mood and alleviate stress.

The Role of Good Genes

While lifestyle habits undoubtedly contribute to the longevity observed in Blue Zones, genetic predispositions also play a role (Caruso, 2022). Some populations in these areas may have genetic factors that make them more resistant to certain diseases or that confer other health advantages.

Sirtuin Genes

A significant area of study involves the sirtuin genes, which regulate critical biological processes including aging and stress resistance. Populations in Blue Zones may have beneficial variants of these genes, helping them combat the negative effects of aging and reducing the risk of chronic diseases such as heart disease and diabetes.

Cholesterol Metabolism

Other genetic factors, such as variations in genes related to cholesterol metabolism, can be more common in Blue Zone populations. Certain genetic profiles lead to lower levels of harmful LDL cholesterol while promoting higher levels of protective HDL cholesterol, reducing heart disease risk.

Telomeres

Telomeres, the protective caps on chromosomes, are also linked to aging. Shorter telomeres are associated with increased aging and disease risk. Individuals in Blue Zones may have genetic traits that help maintain telomere length contributing to healthier aging.

Epigenetics

The interaction between genetics and lifestyle is crucial. For example, diets rich in antioxidants and omega-3 fatty acids can positively influence gene expression related to health and longevity. This relationship, known as epigenetics, shows how lifestyle choices can impact genetic functioning.

While genetics provide advantages, they are not deterministic. The healthy lifestyle habits of Blue Zone residents interact with their genetic makeup to enhance longevity.

Combined Effects of Various Factors Improve Quality of Life

Several examples illustrate how the combined effect of these lifestyle factors contributes to increased lifespan.

Intergenerational Bonds and Nutrient-Rich Diets

Take Okinawa, Japan, one of the most widely studied Blue Zones. The elderly population engages in numerous intergenerational activities, maintaining strong family and community ties. Their diet is primarily composed of sweet potatoes, soy products, vegetables, and fish, all of which are low in calories but nutrient-dense.

Mediterranean Diet, Active Lifestyle, and Relaxation

Similarly, in Ikaria, Greece, another Blue Zone, residents follow a Mediterranean diet and regularly perform physical activities like gardening and walking. They also practice afternoon napping, contributing to their relaxed way of living.

Positive Outlook, Social Bonds, and a Nutrient-Rich Diet

In Costa Rica's Nicoya Peninsula, a positive outlook on life combined with close social networks and a simple, nutrient-rich diet contributes to long life spans. Elderly residents remain active, performing daily chores and participating in community gatherings. Their diet consists of beans, corn, squash, and tropical fruits, which provide the essential nutrients needed for good health.

Active Lifestyles, Nutrient-Rich Diets, and Strong Social Bonds

Sardinia, Italy, offers another compelling case. Men here have some of the highest life expectancies in the world. Their active lifestyle marked by shepherding and farming, ensures they remain physically fit throughout their lives. They enjoy a diet rich in whole grains, vegetables, and lean proteins from sources such as goat's milk and fish. Additionally, Sardinians value strong familial ties and communal living, often coming together for celebrations and daily interactions.

Faith, Vegetarianism, and Community Cohesion for Longevity

Loma Linda, California, showcases how religious beliefs and community cohesion can impact longevity. Many residents are Seventh-day Adventists who follow a vegetarian diet, avoid smoking and alcohol, and emphasize regular physical activity and spiritual well-being. Their faith encourages them to build supportive relationships and engage in charitable acts, which strengthen their social bonds and reduce stress.

Integrating Science and Lifestyle

Spending time near water can significantly reduce stress levels and lead to immediate improvements in mood. Imagine walking along a serene lakeside, listening to the gentle lapping of waves against the shore. This simple act has been shown to lower cortisol levels, the hormone associated with stress.

A reduction in cortisol can result in an overall feeling of relaxation and happiness. Whether it's an afternoon at the beach, a walk by a river, or even just sitting by a fountain, the proximity to water has a calming effect on the mind.

Additionally, engaging in water-based activities goes beyond mere relaxation; it promotes both physical fitness and mental well-being. Swimming is a full-body workout that improves cardiovascular health, builds muscle strength, and increases flexibility. The rhythmic nature of swimming can also serve as a form of meditation, helping to quiet the mind and reduce anxiety.

Kayaking offers a similar blend of physical exertion and mental tranquility. The repetitive paddling motions combined with the natural surroundings create an immersive experience that enhances mental clarity and emotional resilience.

Concluding Thoughts

We explored the various factors contributing to longevity and happiness, with a particular focus on the benefits of water-rich environments. The integration of regular physical activity, nutritious diets, strong social connections, and effective stress management are key components observed in Blue Zones.

These elements work together to create an environment that supports long, healthy lives. Additionally, spending time near bodies of water or engaging in water-based activities can significantly enhance mental well-being by reducing stress levels and promoting relaxation.

By combining scientific findings with practical lifestyle choices, individuals can harness the advantages provided by water-rich environments for both physical and mental health.

Chapter 3:

Subconscious Awareness of Water Proximity

Our subconscious mind perceives the presence of water, a truly fascinating aspect of human sensory and psychological experience. The ability to detect water without consciously realizing it engages various senses and draws on deeply embedded evolutionary adaptations. We will focus on the subtleties of these subconscious processes, highlighting how they influence our interaction with water bodies in ways we might not overtly recognize.

Sensory Input Beyond Sight

Our awareness of water proximity extends beyond the visual realm, tapping into a range of other senses that work subconsciously to detect its presence. When we think about identifying bodies of water, our mind might swiftly conjure up images of serene lakes or crashing ocean waves.

However, several other sensory inputs come into play, often unnoticed by our conscious mind yet instrumental in guiding us toward water sources.

We Can Smell Water

The olfactory system is incredibly sensitive and capable of picking up the distinct scents associated with different types of water bodies. Our sense of smell is one of the most primal senses, deeply connected to our emotions and memories. This sensitivity allows us to perceive the unique aromas that water bodies emit, enhancing our experiences in natural environments.

The Smell of the Beach

Think back to a walk along the beach. The air is often filled with the distinctive saltiness of the sea. This scent is laden with various marine chemicals, including salts and organic compounds released by marine life. As we inhale, these particles travel through the air and are detected by our smell receptors, which then transmit signals to the brain.

The subconscious mind processes these signals rapidly. Before we even set eyes on the ocean, our brain alerts us to its presence, evoking feelings of relaxation and happiness. This innate ability to detect water enhances our connection to the environment and influences our behavior, drawing us closer to the source of this familiar scent.

The Smell of Lakes and Rivers

Freshwater sources, such as lakes and rivers, also have their distinct aromas. These earthy scents are often produced by decaying organic matter and microbial activity in the water. The specific combination of compounds released by plants and microorganisms creates a distinct smell that we can identify, often associated with lush, vibrant ecosystems.

The ability to distinguish between different types of water bodies through scent is not only fascinating but also practical. It enables us to react accordingly, whether it's seeking out the refreshing coolness of a river on a hot day or the calming waves of the ocean.

We Can Hear Water Sources

Sound waves produced by water movement can be powerful indicators of its proximity. Think of the rhythmic sound of crashing waves on the shore or the gentle babbling of a nearby stream. Even when not directly focusing on these noises, our auditory system picks them up and processes them.

Our auditory system is highly attuned to these water-related sounds. Even when we aren't consciously focusing on them, our ears and brain pick up and process these auditory signals. This ability enhances our awareness of our surroundings, allowing us to respond to the presence of water even when it's not directly in our line of sight.

Unconsciously Detecting Water Through Sounds

Interestingly, this detection of water-related sounds often occurs without our conscious realization. Researchers have found that in environments where visual stimuli are limited or absent, individuals can accurately sense the direction and distance of water sources based solely on sound (Song, 2023). This phenomenon highlights our innate connection to nature and the significance of sound as a guide.

Emotions From the Sounds of Water

The sounds of water also evoke a range of emotions. The soothing sound of flowing water can induce relaxation and tranquility, while the powerful crash of ocean waves may inspire awe and respect for nature's force. These auditory experiences enhance our relationship with water bodies.

Using Hearing for Survival

Furthermore, the ability to hear water sources plays a crucial role in survival, especially in natural settings. Recognizing the sounds of water can lead us to essential resources, particularly in wilderness situations where visual cues are scarce. This instinctive skill highlights the remarkable ways our senses work together to navigate the environment.

We Can Feel Nearby Water

Humidity levels also play a significant role in our subconscious detection of water. Proximity to large water bodies often leads to increased moisture in the air. Human skin and respiratory systems respond to varying humidity levels, often more so than we consciously realize.

High humidity can cause slight changes in skin texture and perspiration levels, which our body notices and reacts to instinctively. Additionally, breathing in moist air versus dry air feels different, and our lungs can detect this change. These internal bodily responses are processed by our brain, keeping us subtly aware of water's presence even if we're not actively thinking about it.

Also, large water bodies often influence local atmospheric pressure, creating subtle changes that can affect our senses. When near the sea, for instance, the barometric pressure tends to be slightly lower due to the vast expanse of water.

Though we may not overtly recognize these pressure variations, our inner ear and other pressure-sensitive mechanisms in our body respond to them. It's similar to how some people can feel a storm approaching due to shifts in atmospheric pressure. Over time, our bodies have become attuned to these changes, adding another layer to our subconscious awareness of water nearby.

My Personal Connection to Water

Lake Champlain, which forms the boundary between northern New York and northern Vermont, is not only historically significant but also breathtakingly beautiful. It was the source of my deep connection to water, something I discovered early in life, though I didn't fully realize its influence at the time. Today, and always, Lake Champlain will be my sanctuary on this blue planet.

Although the origin of the quote is uncertain, its essence resonates deeply with me: "Lake Champlain rests between two majestic mountain ranges, offering unparalleled beauty, charm, and serenity."

Long before my yearly return to Burlington, Vermont, I picture the mirror-like perfection of Lake Champlain as the sun rises over the Green Mountains. "Spectacular" doesn't do it justice—it must be experienced. That experience, whether imagined or witnessed, is what truly fuels the essence of Blue Mindedness.

Evolutionary Adaptation and Physiological Changes

The proximity to water is critical in human evolution. Our ancestors relied on water sources for hydration, food, and transportation, making it essential for survival (Rosinger, 2021). This connection may have developed

an inherent sensitivity to the presence of water so deeply
embedded in our subconscious that we react to it even
without conscious awareness.

Relaxing Effects of Water

When people find themselves near bodies of water, they
often report feeling calmer and more at ease. This
reaction may be an evolutionary adaptation.

Water represented safety and sustenance for early
humans; hence, being close to it likely induced a sense of
security and well-being. Over time, these responses
could have been wired into our subconscious, creating a
natural sense of relaxation when we are near water.

Additionally, being around water has been linked to
reduced stress. This phenomenon can be attributed to
the various sensory stimulations provided by water,
including its sound, sight, and even scent.

The visual appeal of water bodies also plays a part. The
vastness of an ocean or the serene stillness of a lake can
captivate our attention, giving our minds a break from
daily stressors.

We Seek Water for Relief

People often seek out vacations by the beach, hikes near
waterfalls, or homes with views of lakes and rivers,
sometimes without fully understanding why. This
instinctual behavior emphasizes our deep-rooted

connection to water and its profound effect on our mental and physiological states.

Water has a significant impact on our mental and physiological states. Spending time near water can reduce stress and enhance mood. The soothing sounds and sights of flowing water help lower anxiety and promote relaxation.

Engaging in water activities such as swimming or lounging by the shore, provides both physical refreshment and emotional relief. These experiences allow us to disconnect from daily stresses, offering a sanctuary for rejuvenation.

Historically, water has been vital for survival, reinforcing our attraction to it. This ancestral connection deepens our instinct to seek water as a source of comfort and well-being. The aesthetics of water bodies also play a role in our attraction. The sight of a sparkling lake or crashing waves can evoke peace and happiness, intensifying our desire to be near water.

Water Therapies

Moreover, therapy practices such as blue space therapy underline the significance of water in managing stress and promoting mental health. These therapies utilize the calming influence of water environments to treat conditions like anxiety and depression.

By bringing patients closer to water, therapists leverage the innate relaxing effects of these settings, offering a tangible example of how subconscious responses to water can be harnessed for positive outcomes (Hydrotherapy and Mental Health: Therapeutic Benefits of Water, n.d.).

The following are examples of soothing water therapies:

Hydrotherapy

Hydrotherapy involves the use of water for pain relief and treatment. Techniques include whirlpool baths, cold packs, and warm compresses, which can help alleviate muscle and joint pain, improve circulation, and promote relaxation.

Aquatic Therapy

Conducted in a warm water pool, this therapy uses the properties of water to facilitate physical rehabilitation. Patients engage in exercises designed to improve strength, flexibility, and balance, making it particularly beneficial for those with arthritis or mobility issues.

Watsu

A form of bodywork that combines elements of shiatsu and floating in warm water. Practitioners gently support and move clients through the water, promoting deep relaxation, reducing stress, and relieving muscle tension.

Floatation Therapy

This involves lying in a sensory deprivation tank filled with highly salted water, allowing for buoyancy and relaxation. This therapy helps reduce anxiety, stress, and chronic pain by creating a weightless environment that minimizes external stimuli.

Saltwater Therapy (Halotherapy)

Saltwater therapy involves inhaling salt-infused air in a controlled environment, often mimicking the conditions of a salt mine or the beach. It is thought to help with respiratory issues, skin conditions, and overall relaxation.

Considering all these, it is evident that our interactions with water go beyond mere necessity. They are embedded in our biology and psychology. Recognizing the importance of this connection can lead to better mental health practices and a deeper appreciation for natural water bodies in our surroundings.

Final Insights

We learned the fascinating ways our subconscious mind can sense and respond to the presence of water. Through a combination of olfactory, auditory, and tactile inputs, we can detect water sources without our conscious awareness.

Understanding these sensory mechanisms highlights the profound impact of water on our well-being. The feelings of calm and relaxation experienced near water are not merely coincidental but are ingrained in our physiology.

Chapter 4:

Community and

Connection in Blue Spaces

Blue spaces promote community building and social interaction. Let's examine the role of social networks in providing emotional and practical support, contributing significantly to overall well-being. We will explore how inclusivity and accessibility in these environments can foster a sense of belonging, creating resilient and contented communities.

Social Fabric of Blue Zones

In Blue Zones, communities demonstrate higher levels of social interaction, communal activities, and shared spaces. These regions offer settings that naturally encourage people to come together. Whether it's through group fishing outings, communal gardening by the water's edge, or neighborhood gatherings on the beach, the act of sharing these blue spaces fosters a sense of camaraderie and unity.

This interaction is not just about physical proximity; it extends into deep social bonds that are formed as individuals engage in collective activities.

Reduces Stress Levels and Increases Satisfaction

The strong sense of belonging in Blue Zones plays a vital role in reducing stress levels and increasing life satisfaction. In these communities, people feel deeply connected to those around them, which provides emotional stability and security.

Being part of a community offers a psychological anchor, giving individuals a sense of purpose and meaning. This connection lowers anxiety, as people feel valued, understood, and supported by those around them.

A strong sense of belonging also helps reduce mental fatigue. Knowing they are part of something larger than themselves can be incredibly comforting, offering both relief and empowerment.

Contributes to Longevity and Mental Health

The practice of "Moai" in Okinawa, Japan is an example of this, where groups of friends commit to supporting each other throughout their lives. These groups meet regularly, share experiences, and provide mutual assistance, which cultivates strong social ties and has been linked to the remarkable longevity of Okinawans.

Similarly, in Sardinia, Italy, elderly residents gather frequently to share meals and stories, strengthening intergenerational bonds. These community practices are not just social engagements; they are integral to the way of life that promotes health and longevity.

Promotes Healthier Lifestyles

A community that values outdoor activities and fresh, locally sourced food will likely see its members adopting these habits, leading to better health outcomes.

Emotional well-being is also closely tied to these community interactions. In Blue Zones, people discuss their problems openly with friends and receive practical advice and empathy. This helps mitigate stress and fosters a balanced, optimistic outlook on life.

Creating Blue Zone Communities in Blue Mind Environments

Fostering a sense of community around water involves organizing events and groups that facilitate bonding and interaction. Hosting gatherings or meet-ups at local water spots is an excellent way to bring people together.

Casual Meet-Ups Near Water

Imagine a sunny afternoon at the local beach where families, friends, and even strangers can come together to share a picnic, play beach volleyball, or simply enjoy the waves. Such informal gatherings create a welcoming environment where people feel comfortable connecting with others.

Beach Gatherings

To organize a casual beach meet-up, one option is to host a community picnic. Invite people to bring blankets, snacks, and drinks, and set up near the shoreline. This laid-back setup encourages mingling, sharing food, and exchanging stories. Adding a game of beach volleyball or frisbee can engage groups and build friendly competition, creating teamwork and camaraderie.

Waterfront Bonfires

Whether at the beach or by a lake, bonfires offer a cozy setting where people can gather, roast marshmallows, and chat as the sun sets. The warmth of the fire and the sound of waves in the background create an inviting atmosphere for relaxation and storytelling.

Active Gatherings

For a more active gathering, consider organizing a kayaking or paddleboarding group. Renting equipment and setting off on a leisurely paddle along the water encourages participants to interact and enjoy the natural surroundings. It is a fun way to explore new areas while bonding with others who share similar interests.

Community Clean-Ups

Community clean-up events near water can bring people together with a shared sense of purpose. Volunteers can work together to clean up litter from beaches, rivers, or lakes, fostering a sense of community pride and connection to the environment. Afterward, participants can relax together with a picnic or refreshments, celebrating their collective efforts.

By creating opportunities for casual, water-based meet-ups, people are more likely to form lasting connections, reduce stress, and enjoy the sense of community that naturally arises in these beautiful settings.

Water-Focused Groups or Clubs

Joining or creating local clubs focused on water-based activities can foster regular social engagement and a stronger sense of community. These groups not only promote physical well-being but also provide a structured way for members to connect regularly, share experiences, and enjoy water-related activities together.

Kayaking Club

Starting a kayaking club is a great way to bring people together who share a love for adventure and the outdoors. Organize regular outings to local lakes, rivers, or the coast where members can paddle, explore different waterways, and socialize. Each outing could include a picnic or a group discussion about paddling techniques and the best local spots to kayak, fostering deeper connections over shared experiences.

Beach Walking Group

Another option is a beach walking group, which offers a more relaxed, low-impact activity for all ages. Members could meet early in the morning to walk along the shoreline, enjoying the peaceful sounds of the waves and the calming atmosphere. After the walk, the group could stop at a local cafe for coffee, encouraging further social interaction and bonding. This type of group is not only great for fitness but also for starting the day with fresh air and friendly conversation.

Water Aerobics Club

For those who enjoy swimming, a water aerobics club at a community pool or natural body of water can be a great idea. Regular sessions with different routines, such as aqua yoga or low-impact water workouts, offer a way for members to stay active while engaging socially. After each session, participants can gather to chat, sharing tips and stories that strengthen camaraderie.

Paddleboarding Session

Hosting a weekly paddleboarding session can also bring together water enthusiasts. Members could meet at a local river or beach for a session, taking turns helping newcomers learn balance and paddling techniques. Paddleboarding is a social sport, and after a session, the group can gather on the shore for snacks and casual conversation, deepening friendships and encouraging more participation.

Water Conservation Group

For those focused on environmental initiatives, starting a water conservation group that engages in activities like beach cleanups, water quality testing, or advocacy for protecting local water bodies is a meaningful way to connect with others. The group could organize events to raise awareness, participate in workshops, or plan recreational outings as a reward for their efforts.

Online Platforms

Online platforms or social media can be used to organize water-focused groups making it easy to communicate, plan events, and encourage new members to join. By creating consistent opportunities for members to meet and interact around water-based activities, these clubs foster a strong sense of community, friendships, and shared passion.

Educational Workshops

Workshops on marine conservation or guided tours exploring local aquatic flora and fauna can be both informative and socially engaging. These activities provide a platform for learning and discussion, sparking conversations that can lead to deeper connections. They also attract like-minded individuals who share a passion for the environment, further solidifying the community's bond.

Marine Conservation Workshop

Organizing marine conservation workshops that cover topics such as pollution, coral reef protection, and sustainable fishing practices can inspire meaningful dialogue. Participants can engage in hands-on activities such as water testing or shoreline clean-ups that make the learning experience interactive and foster teamwork. After the event, informal discussions over lunch or coffee can deepen relationships as participants reflect on what they've learned and share personal experiences related to environmental activism.

Guided Tours

A guided tour of local rivers, lakes, or coastal areas to explore aquatic flora and fauna is another way to encourage both education and socializing. Local biologists or conservationists could lead the tours, explaining the significance of various plant and animal species in the ecosystem. After the tour, group discussions can help reinforce learning while also offering a relaxed setting for participants to bond over their shared interest in nature.

Water-Focused Lectures

Water-focused lecture series invites experts to speak on topics such as marine biodiversity, water conservation efforts, or climate change's impact on aquatic life. These workshops can be followed by Q and A sessions where attendees can ask questions and share their views. The discussions that emerge can spark lasting connections between people who are passionate about the environment.

DIY Conservation Projects

Workshops can include DIY conservation projects, where participants create things like rainwater collection systems, wildlife-friendly gardens, or recycled water filters. These collaborative projects not only educate people but also provide a shared goal, creating stronger bonds within the group as they work together for a cause.

To encourage broader participation, these educational workshops can be advertised through local schools, libraries, or online community forums. Hosting follow-up events, such as social gatherings or eco-friendly outdoor activities, can maintain engagement and keep connections alive.

Kids' Programs

Children's programs, such as summer camps focused on water safety and aquatic sports, can also contribute significantly to community building. These programs allow kids to make new friends and build teamwork skills in a fun and supportive setting. Parents, too, benefit from these activities as they meet and connect with other families, creating a network of support and camaraderie.

Water Safety Camp

A water safety camp could teach kids how to swim, how to respond to water emergencies, and the importance of respecting natural water bodies. Through engaging activities such as swimming lessons, lifesaving drills, and interactive games, children build confidence in the water while bonding with peers. The friendships formed in this environment often extend beyond camp, creating long-lasting social connections.

Aquatic Sports Programs

Programs such as canoeing, paddleboarding, or junior sailing, allow kids to explore new hobbies while working together in teams. These activities promote cooperation, problem-solving, and leadership skills. Team-based competitions or group challenges can further strengthen bonds as children work together to achieve common goals.

Meet and Connect

Parents also benefit from these programs as they have the opportunity to meet and connect with other families during drop-offs, pick-ups, and camp events. These interactions create a network of support, where parents can share advice, arrange playdates, or collaborate on community activities. By organizing family-friendly events such as parent-kid relay races or a family beach day, these programs can encourage deeper interaction between families, fostering camaraderie.

Educational Water Safety Workshops

Hosting educational water safety workshops for parents alongside the kids' programs can provide additional value. Parents learn how to keep their children safe around water while also connecting with other caregivers who share similar concerns and experiences.

Advertise these kids' programs through local schools, community centers, or online platforms. This ensures families from different backgrounds can participate and engage. By bringing families together around water-based activities, these programs help build a stronger, more interconnected community, where both children and parents benefit socially and emotionally.

Consider Inclusivity

Inclusivity is another essential aspect of fostering community around blue spaces. Ensuring that events and activities are accessible to everyone, including those with disabilities or limited mobility, can make a significant difference.

Accessible Amenities

This might include ramps for easy access to water, ensuring beaches, lakesides, or docks are navigable for those using wheelchairs or other mobility devices. Offering accessible watercraft such as adaptive kayaks or paddleboards can allow individuals with different abilities to participate in aquatic activities without barriers. Additionally, make sure there are designated parking spots and clear paths from parking areas to the water to ensure everyone, regardless of mobility, can comfortably enjoy water-based events.

Inclusive Opportunities

Inclusivity also extends to creating opportunities for individuals of all ages, backgrounds, and fitness levels to participate. For example, offering a variety of activities, from more physically demanding options such as swimming or kayaking to gentler activities such as birdwatching near the water or fishing from an accessible dock, ensures everyone can find something they enjoy.

Inclusive Programming

Creating inclusive programming such as family-friendly events, multi-generational activities, or special accommodations for individuals with sensory sensitivities, helps foster a sense of belongingness. These efforts also encourage interactions that further enrich community bonds.

The goal of fostering community around water through organized events and groups is to create lasting relationships and a collective sense of belonging. These efforts can transform blue spaces into vibrant hubs of social activity, where individuals come together to enjoy, protect, and celebrate their natural surroundings.

Water Has Shaped My Life, My Journey

Throughout my life, I've always lived near a significant body of water, whether by intention or some subconscious pull. Water has been my constant magnet—Lake Champlain in Burlington, VT, with its serene and expansive beauty; the Atlantic Ocean in Virginia Beach, VA, where powerful waves meet endless shores; the warm, tranquil waters of the Gulf of Mexico in Sarasota, FL; the stunning Pacific Ocean in San Diego, CA, with its dramatic coastline and endless horizons; and the crystal-clear, picturesque beaches of the Mediterranean Sea in Barcelona, Spain.

Water has shaped my journey, connecting each place I've called home. No matter where I go, it remains my anchor and source of inspiration.

Final Thoughts

We learned the significance of Blue Zones and the unique ways these water-centric environments foster a strong sense of community and social connection. The positive impact of shared water-based activities on both physical and mental health is clear. These activities promote fitness and strengthen social ties through shared experiences.

Organized events and clubs provide consistent opportunities for interaction, fostering enduring friendships and a robust community spirit. Integration of blue spaces into our lives offers a pathway to a healthier, happier, and more connected society.

Chapter 5:

Purpose and Blue Mindful Living

Having a clear sense of purpose is an integral factor in uniting Blue Zones. Whether through individual reflection, community involvement, or creating personal rituals, let us uncover ways to harness the power of purpose and water to achieve a more fulfilling and healthier existence.

Purpose in Blue Zones

Having a life purpose significantly influences one's longevity and overall well-being. When we talk about purpose, we delve into what gets us out of bed in the morning with enthusiasm and what drives our actions throughout the day.

Research and studies have shown that individuals who possess a clear sense of purpose tend to live longer and healthier lives (Berman, 2022). This isn't merely a correlation but one intertwined with various physiological and psychological benefits.

The Science Behind Purpose

From a biological perspective, having a sense of purpose can lead to lower levels of stress and inflammation, both of which are known to contribute to chronic diseases. When you have goals and aspirations, your body releases beneficial hormones like endorphins, also known as "feel-good" hormones.

These hormones improve your mood and help reduce anxiety, making you feel more positive. However, the benefits go beyond that. Endorphins also boost immunity, making it easier for the body to fight illness.

Additionally, having a sense of purpose can improve your sleep quality. When you're less stressed and have fulfilling goals, you're more likely to sleep well. Good sleep is important because it helps your body recover and keeps your mind sharp. Better sleep patterns not only support your physical health but also improve your memory and cognitive function.

Having a Purpose Encourages Positive Behaviors

Purpose encourages proactive behaviors, such as regular exercise, healthy eating, and routine medical check-ups, which are crucial for longevity. People who believe their lives have meaning are more likely to take care of themselves because they see value in staying healthy.

One compelling example comes from the Blue Zones— regions of the world where people live significantly longer than average. In these areas, having a purpose, also known as "ikigai" in Okinawa, Japan is a common thread among centenarians.

These individuals don't just live long; they live well, filled with engagement, joy, and connection. They awake each day with a clear intent, whether it's tending to a garden, spending time with grandchildren, or contributing to their community.

Defining Your Purpose Through Mindfulness

Incorporating mindfulness practices can greatly assist in this journey. Mindfulness allows us to stay present and attuned to our experiences, helping us identify what truly resonates with us.

Here are mindfulness activities to help you define your purpose.

Meditation for Clarity

Spend 10-15 minutes each day practicing mindful meditation. Sit quietly, close your eyes, and focus on your breath. When your mind starts to wander, gently guide it back to your breathing. Over time, this practice clears mental clutter, allowing you to reflect on what truly matters in your life and helping you discover your deeper purpose.

Journaling Your Thoughts

Set aside time to journal your thoughts, feelings, and experiences daily or weekly. Write freely about your passions, things that make you feel fulfilled, and moments where you feel the most connected to yourself. Reflect on these entries regularly, patterns may emerge that point you to your core values and sense of purpose.

Purposeful Walking

Take a mindful walk in nature or around your neighborhood, fully focusing on your surroundings. Pay attention to the sounds, sights, and smells as you walk. Use this time to reflect on your goals, aspirations, and what brings you joy. Walking with intention can spark new insights and help align your purpose with your daily life.

Visualization Exercises

Try visualization to imagine your ideal future. Picture yourself living a life filled with meaning and purpose. What does that look like? What are you doing, and how are you impacting others? This mental exercise can provide clear guidance on what you want to pursue and what you value most.

Every day, take a few moments to list three things you are grateful for. As you build this gratitude habit, notice the recurring themes—things that consistently bring joy and fulfillment. Identifying what you appreciate can help you focus on what gives your life meaning, clarifying your purpose over time.

Understanding the importance of purpose doesn't mean every moment must be filled with profound significance. Life's smaller joys and routine tasks also play a pivotal role in our overall sense of well-being. Balancing big-picture goals with daily pleasures creates a harmonious life rhythm, where both ambition and contentment coexist.

Finding Purpose Through Water

Engaging in water-related activities can add depth and meaning to our lives, fostering a profound sense of purpose. Whether by spending reflective moments by the shore or actively participating in conservation efforts, these interactions with water have the potential to transform our mental state and overall well-being.

Have a Specific Intention in Mind

Spend time near water with the intention of reflecting on your life goals; use the calming influence of water to brainstorm new directions or reinforce existing ones. The rhythmic sound of waves, the gentle lapping of a lake, or even the serene flow of a river can create an ideal backdrop for introspection.

- **Set a clear goal beforehand**. Before heading to the water, identify what you want to reflect on—whether it's your career, relationships, or personal growth. This gives your thoughts direction and helps you stay focused.

- **Choose the right water setting.** Pick a water body that matches your mood. A peaceful lake may be best for deep thinking while the energy of the waves or flowing water could help boost your creativity. Consider the setting that will help enhance the reflection process.

- **Incorporate breathing exercises.** While near water, use deep breathing exercises to center yourself. Synchronize your breath with the rhythm of the waves or flowing water. This not only calms your mind but also helps open up your thoughts for new insights.

- **Use water sounds for guided meditation.** Bring along a guided meditation track focused on goal-setting or personal growth. The natural sounds of water can amplify the meditative experience and help you visualize your goals more clearly.

Engage in Purposeful Tasks

Volunteering for coastal clean-ups or water conservation efforts helps preserve vital ecosystems and instills a sense of achievement and contribution. These activities provide a dual benefit: they address environmental issues while simultaneously offering participants a fulfilling experience.

Here are tips to help you make your involvement in these activities more impactful.

- **Research local environmental needs.** Before volunteering, learn about the specific challenges in the area. Whether it's coastal erosion, pollution, or endangered marine species, understanding the local issues helps you focus your efforts where they are most needed.

- **Join or start a group.** Consider joining a local environmental organization or starting your own group for regular clean-ups or water conservation initiatives. Being part of a community amplifies your impact and allows you to engage with like-minded individuals.

- **Set personal goals for each activity.** When participating in a clean-up or conservation effort, set small personal goals such as collecting a certain amount of trash or planting a specific number of trees. These goals can provide a sense of accomplishment and drive your motivation.

- **Reflect on the impact.** After each task, take time to reflect on the difference you've made and how it contributes to the bigger picture. This reflection can reinforce your sense of purpose and motivate you to continue participating in environmental efforts.

Choose Meaningful Water Activities

Swimming, kayaking, or even paddleboarding can also become meaningful experiences when approached with mindfulness and intention. These are also opportunities to connect with nature and oneself. The focus required during these activities helps cultivate a presence of mind that translates into other areas of life. When individuals are fully engaged in such pursuits, they often find themselves more grounded and aware, reinforcing their sense of purpose and well-being.

Here are tips to enhance your experience and reinforce your sense of purpose.

- **Set an intention for each activity.** Before starting your water activity, take a moment to set a specific intention. Whether it's to practice gratitude, enjoy the moment, or reflect on personal goals, having a clear purpose can deepen your connection to the experience.

- **Practice mindful movement.** Focus on the sensations in your body as you engage in your chosen activity. Feel the water against your skin, listen to the sounds around you, and observe the beauty of your surroundings. This mindfulness can help you cultivate a greater sense of presence and awareness.

- **Incorporate breathwork.** Use your breath as a tool to enhance your experience. For example, while swimming, synchronize your breathing with your strokes. In kayaking or paddleboarding, take deep, calming breaths as you navigate the water, promoting relaxation and clarity of mind.

- **Capture the experience.** Bring a waterproof camera or journal to document your adventures. Taking photos or writing about your experiences can help you reflect on your time spent on the water, reinforcing the meaningful moments and insights gained during these activities.

Incorporate Water Rituals

Simple practices such as starting the day with a meditative walk by the beach or ending it with a relaxing bath can become powerful anchors in one's schedule. These rituals serve as reminders of the tranquility and clarity that water brings, helping individuals maintain a balanced and focused mindset amidst life's challenges.

The following are tips to integrate water rituals into your life.

- **Morning meditative walks:** Begin your day with a peaceful walk by a lake, river, or ocean. Use this time to focus on your breath, observe the surroundings, and set a positive intention for the day ahead. The combination of fresh air and the calming presence of water can invigorate your spirit.

- **Gratitude rituals:** After your water activities, take a moment to express gratitude. Reflect on the beauty of the water, your experiences, and what you appreciate in life. This simple practice can help cultivate a positive mindset and enhance your overall well-being.

- **Evening relaxation baths:** End your day with a soothing bath infused with essential oils and bath salts. Use this time to unwind and reflect on the day's events. Consider adding calming music or soft candlelight to create a serene atmosphere that enhances relaxation.

- **Weekly water reflection time:** Dedicate time each week to reflect by water. This could be sitting by a pond, visiting a local beach, or even a backyard fountain. Bring a journal to jot down thoughts, feelings, and insights that arise during this reflective time.

Encourage Children to Join Water-Related Activities

Teaching them to swim, snorkel, or fish can lay the foundation for a meaningful relationship with water. As they grow, these early experiences can evolve into broader environmental awareness and a commitment to conservation efforts. By fostering this connection early on, parents and educators can instill values of stewardship and purpose in future generations.

- **Enroll in swim lessons:** Start with basic swimming lessons at an early age. Look for local swim classes that focus on safety and technique, allowing children to build confidence in the water. Mastering swimming also opens doors to other water activities.

- **Organize family outings:** Plan regular family trips to lakes, rivers, or beaches. Engage in activities like picnicking, beachcombing, or simply playing in the water. These outings create memorable experiences and help children appreciate the beauty and joy that water can bring.

- **Explore snorkeling and fishing:** Introduce children to snorkeling in calm, shallow waters where they can observe marine life. Additionally, teach them fishing techniques, emphasizing patience and the thrill of catching their own food.

- **Create water-themed crafts and activities:** Encourage creativity by incorporating water themes into arts and crafts. For instance, children can create fish models, make ocean-themed collages, or engage in science experiments related to water. These activities can reinforce their understanding of aquatic environments and the importance of conservation.

Water's role in cultural and spiritual practices worldwide underscores its universal significance. Exploring how different communities celebrate and honor water can add a rich layer of meaning to one's own water-related practices.

My First Experience With Water

My earliest memory of Lake Champlain is from when my mother took me to Cliffside Park for swim lessons. I was about four or five years old. As the instructor led me into the water, with my mother nearby, I began to scream—I was terrified. I didn't know why, perhaps because the water was dark and cold. Even now, I cannot explain my fear, as I recall nothing that should have caused it. I didn't learn to swim that day; after swallowing water when told to put my head under, the lesson ended.

I eventually overcame my fear. Our family spent every summer weekend at a camp on the lake, and one day, one of my seven older sisters taught me the dog paddle. With that simple stroke, my fear vanished, and my confidence grew. That summer, over sixty years ago, marked the beginning of my love for the lake.

Final Thoughts

We examined the profound impact of having a life purpose and engaging in water-related activities on longevity and mindfulness. Purpose can reduce stress, boost immune function, and enhance mental well-being.

Water-related activities are effective means to foster purpose and mindfulness. Whether through reflective moments by the shore, active participation in conservation efforts, or engaging in sports like swimming and kayaking, spending time near water enhances clarity and connection to one's goals. Simple daily rituals involving water can provide tranquility and balance, reinforcing one's purpose and well-being in everyday life.

Chapter 6

Movement and Water-Inspired Activities

Various forms of natural movements contribute to physical health. We will focus on the benefits of water-based activities gaining insights into how these practices improve physical health and offer substantial mental health benefits. Learn practical ways to integrate both land and water-inspired activities into your lifestyles, promoting a holistic approach to well-being.

Movement in Blue Zones: Natural, Low-Intensity Daily Physical Activities

Understanding the lifestyle practices of Blue Zones provides invaluable insights. In these regions, residents incorporate natural, low intensity daily physical activities into their routines.

A key aspect of life in Blue Zones is the integration of movement into daily tasks. Unlike structured exercise regimens common in many parts of the world, physical activity in Blue Zones is an organic part of everyday life. Let's examine the most common activities of residents in these places.

Walking

Whether it's commuting to work, visiting friends, or running errands, walking is a fundamental aspect of daily routines. Walking increases overall physical activity and promotes cardiovascular health by ensuring the heart works moderately but consistently enhancing endurance and lowering the risk of heart-related diseases.

Follow these tips to use walking as an activity for wellness.

- **Incorporate walking into daily routines:** Make walking a regular part of your day by opting for it instead of driving for short trips. Walk to school, work, or nearby shops. This not only increases your physical activity but also adds a refreshing break to your daily tasks.

- **Schedule social walks:** Turn walks into social events by inviting friends or family to join you. Walking with others can boost motivation and make the experience enjoyable. Consider organizing weekly walking meet-ups in your local park or neighborhood.

- **Explore nature trails:** Seek out local nature trails, parks, or waterfront paths for your walks. Being in a natural environment enhances the calming effects of walking and can improve mental well-being. Take time to observe your surroundings, listen to the sounds of nature, and breathe in the fresh air.

- **Practice mindful walking:** Use your walking time to practice mindfulness. Focus on your breath, the rhythm of your steps, and the sensations in your body. This practice helps clear your mind, reduce stress, and increase your overall awareness of the present moment.

- **Set walking goals:** Aim to set achievable walking goals, such as walking a specific number of steps each day or exploring new routes. Tracking your progress with a pedometer or a mobile app can keep you motivated and help you celebrate your achievements.

Gardening

Gardening combines light aerobic exercise with muscle-strengthening tasks, such as digging, planting, and weeding. Gardening involves both physical exertion and a connection to nature, which can boost mental well-being. The repetitive motions involved in gardening enhance flexibility and strength while providing a tranquil environment that fosters mindfulness and reduces stress.

- **Start small and plan:** If you're new to gardening, begin with a small plot or less number of pots. Choose easy-to-grow plants like herbs and flowers. Planning your garden layout can also provide a sense of purpose and satisfaction as you see your designs come to life.

- **Incorporate regular routine:** Make gardening a regular part of your week. Set aside dedicated time for planting, weeding, or harvesting. This routine not only increases physical activity but also offers a refreshing break from daily stressors.

- **Engage in mindful gardening:** Use gardening as an opportunity for mindfulness. Focus on the textures of the soil, the scents of the plants, and the sounds of nature around you. This can help cultivate a sense of peace and presence, enhancing your well-being.

- **Include family and friends:** Invite family and friends to join you in gardening. Whether it's starting a community garden or simply planting together in your backyard, shared experiences foster connection and make the activity more enjoyable.

- **Celebrate your harvest:** Enjoy the fruits of your labor by incorporating fresh produce from your garden into meals. Cooking with homegrown ingredients adds nutritional value to your diet and reinforces a rewarding feeling of nurturing and growing your own food.

Manual Tasks

From chopping wood to carrying groceries, these chores require physical effort that keeps the body active and engaged. Such tasks often involve various muscle groups, promoting all-around strength and dexterity without the need for deliberate workout sessions.

The rhythm and regularity of these activities ensure that individuals remain physically fit over the long term, mitigating the risks associated with sedentary lifestyles. Consider these tips to transform daily tasks into wellness activities.

- **Prioritize household chores:** Incorporate household chores such as vacuuming, mopping, or tidying up into your routine. These activities provide a great way to keep moving every day. Set a timer and see how much you can accomplish within a specific timeframe to make it more engaging.

- **Combine tasks with intent:** When doing manual tasks, such as carrying groceries or gardening, focus on the physical effort involved. Be mindful of your posture and movements. This awareness can enhance your core strength and flexibility while making the activity more enjoyable.

- **Engage in outdoor manual work:** Take on outdoor projects such as landscaping, yard work, or DIY home improvements. These activities allow you to connect with nature while providing a solid workout. Invite family members or friends to make it a fun group effort.

- **Set goals for manual activities:** Challenge yourself with goals related to manual tasks, such as aiming to chop a certain amount of firewood or carrying a set weight of groceries. Setting and achieving these goals can boost your motivation and provide a sense of accomplishment.

- **Incorporate variety:** Mix up your manual tasks to keep things interesting. Rotate between different chores, such as cooking, cleaning, and gardening. This variety prevents boredom and engages different muscle groups, enhancing overall fitness and well-being.

Mental Benefits of Physical Activities

Beyond physical benefits, engaging in regular, low-intensity activities fosters a sense of purpose and community. The act of walking to a neighbor's house or attending communal gardening projects strengthens social bonds and creates a support network.

These are crucial in mental health, offering emotional support and reducing feelings of loneliness and isolation. In Blue Zones, the emphasis on community and shared activities contributes to a greater sense of belonging and satisfaction with life.

For people inspired by the Blue Zone lifestyle, integrating similar practices into their routine can be straightforward and effective. Starting the day with a brisk walk, engaging in gardening, or choosing manual tasks over automated ones can make a considerable difference. Here are some ideas to inspire you:

- **Start with a daily walk:** Dedicate time each morning or evening for a brisk walk around your neighborhood. This simple activity can boost your mood, provide a sense of purpose, and enhance your connection with nature and your community.

- **Join a community garden:** Get involved in a local gardening project. This promotes physical activity and fosters social connections and collaboration with like-minded individuals.

- **Volunteer for local clean-ups:** Participate in community clean-up days at parks or beaches. This combines physical exertion with environmental stewardship, allowing you to connect with others while making a positive impact.

- **Organize social gatherings:** Host casual meet-ups, such as potlucks or picnics that encourage movement. Play games, go on hikes, or enjoy the outdoors. These gatherings strengthen social ties and enhance feelings of belonging.

- **Incorporate movement into daily tasks:** Choose manual tasks such as gardening, cleaning, or DIY projects over automated options. You can keep physically active and also enjoy opportunities for mindfulness and a sense of accomplishment.

Creating opportunities for movement within daily schedules can transform passive habits into active ones, gradually building a healthier and more dynamic lifestyle.

Benefits of Water-Based Movement: Physical and Mental Health Benefits of Aquatic Exercises

Water-based activities offer unique and effective ways to incorporate physical exercise into daily life. These activities provide comprehensive workouts that engage multiple muscle groups minus the high-impact stress associated with land-based exercises. This makes aquatic exercises suitable for individuals of all ages and fitness levels. Let's look at the best activities to engage in.

Swimming and Aqua Aerobics Are Great Forms of Exercise

The rhythmic movements involved in different strokes work the arms, legs, and core and enhance coordination. Aqua aerobics follows a similar principle, using the resistance of water to increase the intensity of movements while maintaining a low impact on the joints. Here are some tips to make the most of these aquatic exercises:

- **Set clear goals:** Determine what you want to achieve with your routines whether it's improving endurance, building strength, or enhancing flexibility. Setting specific goals can keep you motivated and track your progress.

- **Incorporate variety:** Mix different swimming strokes (freestyle, breaststroke, backstroke, and butterfly) and acquire aerobics routines to engage various muscle groups and prevent boredom. Changing up your workouts can also help you improve overall fitness and keep you challenged.

- **Focus on technique:** Pay attention to your form while swimming or performing aqua aerobics. Proper technique enhances efficiency, reduces the risk of injury, and maximizes the benefits of each movement. Consider taking lessons or watching instructional videos to refine your skills.

- **Stay hydrated:** Drink water before, during, and after your workout to maintain optimum hydration levels and support overall performance.

- **Listen to your body:** Pay attention to how your body feels during and after workouts. Adjust the intensity and duration based on your fitness level and energy. If you're new to swimming or aqua aerobics, start slowly and gradually increase the intensity to prevent overexertion.

Buoyancy Prevents Strain on the Body

Buoyancy significantly reduces the strain on joints, making water activities an excellent choice for individuals with arthritis or those recovering from injuries. The support offered by water allows for a greater range of motion than what might be possible on land, enabling participants to perform a variety of movements with ease and comfort.

Mental Health Benefits

Engaging in aquatic exercises offers profound mental health benefits, as the soothing properties of water create a calming environment that significantly reduces stress and anxiety. The gentle buoyancy of water allows for a sense of weightlessness, which can enhance relaxation and promote a meditative state.

Activities such as swimming or floatation enable you to focus on breathing and body movements supporting mindfulness and encouraging a deep connection to the present movement. This tranquil experience serves as a refreshing escape from stress and restores mental clarity and emotional balance.

Integrate Physical Activities in Your Daily Routines

To maximize the benefits of aquatic exercises, it's advisable to integrate them into a balanced fitness routine. Replace one workout a week with a water-based exercise like swimming, aqua aerobics, or paddleboarding. This change not only diversifies your fitness regimen but also ensures that different muscle groups are engaged in various ways, promoting overall body strength and flexibility.

The Day My Mind Turned Blue

My first boat ride to Juniper Island was in 1960 or '61, and all I remember is how long the trip seemed—it felt endless in "kid time." Today, boats are faster, and the trip is brief. Once you're on the water, though, time seems to disappear—or you simply stop caring. That's the magic of it.

That escape from solid ground shifts your perspective, turning your mind blue, and you realize exactly why you're there.

Final Thoughts

Integrating natural, low-intensity daily physical activities and water-based exercises into our routines can significantly enhance overall well-being. Following the lifestyle practices of Blue Zones, where movement is a seamless part of daily tasks, these help maintain physical and mental health.

Activities such as walking, gardening, and manual tasks incorporate consistent, mild exercise that supports cardiovascular health, muscle strength, and metabolic function. These movements help prevent diseases linked to inactivity while also fostering a sense of community and mental clarity.

Chapter 7:

Diet, Hydration, and the Healing Power of Water

Diet and hydration are fundamental to achieving optimal health and enhancing longevity in Blue Zones. This chapter explores the dietary principles observed in Blue Zones, including the emphasis on plant-based foods and the inclusion of aquatic foods. We will uncover the benefits of avoiding processed foods and the importance of proper hydration.

Blue Zones Diet Principles and Aquatic Foods for Longevity

Blue Zones emphasize a diet that is both sustainable and nutritionally rich. The primary principles revolve around plant-based foods, minimally processed foods, and occasional meat consumption.

Plant-Based Nutrition

Residents consume a variety of whole grains, legumes, vegetables, and fruits daily. Whole grains like oats, barley, brown rice, and whole wheat provide a steady source of energy and are full of fiber, which aids in digestion and helps control blood sugar levels.

Legumes such as beans, lentils, and chickpeas are essential protein sources and contain numerous vitamins and minerals beneficial to overall health. These foods are inexpensive, versatile, and can be incorporated into various dishes to enhance both flavor and nutritional value.

Here are a few techniques to incorporate plant-based nutrition into your diet:

- **Start gradually:** Introduce plant-based meals slowly. Begin with one or two meatless days each week, gradually increasing as you become more comfortable with plant-based options.

- **Explore whole grains:** Experiment with different whole grains such as quinoa, farro, or brown rice. Use them as a base for salads, bowls, or stir-fries to boost nutrition and add variety to your meals.

- **Incorporate more legumes:** Add beans, lentils, or chickpeas to soups, stews, and salads. They are excellent sources of protein and fiber, making meals hearty and satisfying.

- **Embrace seasonal vegetables and fruits:** Fill your plate with a colorful array of seasonal produce. Visit local farmer's markets to discover new fruits and veggies and try new recipes that highlight these ingredients.

Incorporating these tips can help you smoothly transition to a more plant-based diet that enhances your health and well-being.

Vegetables and Fruits

Vegetables and fruits enrich the diet with vitamins, minerals, and antioxidants. They support immune function, reduce inflammation, and protect against chronic diseases.

Leafy greens, cruciferous vegetables (like broccoli and cauliflower), berries, and citrus fruits stand out for their health-promoting properties. Regularly consuming a colorful array of produce ensures that one gets a broad spectrum of nutrients.

Consider these tips to incorporate more vegetables and fruits into your daily meals.

- **Add vegetables to every meal:** Make it a habit to include at least one vegetable in every meal. Whether it's adding spinach to your morning smoothie, including peppers in your omelet, or tossing extra veggies into your stir-fry, these simple steps boost nutrient intake.

- **Snack on fruits and veggies:** Keep cut-up fruits and veggies handy for quick snacks. Carrot sticks, cucumber slices, apple wedges, or berries are easy to grab and can satisfy cravings while providing essential nutrients.

- **Experiment with smoothies:** Blend a variety of fruits and leafy greens into smoothies. This is a delicious way to consume multiple servings of produce at once. Try combinations like bananas with spinach or berries with kale.

- **Make salads a staple:** Create colorful salads using a mix of greens, vegetables, nuts, and seeds. Try different dressings and toppings to keep it exciting. Adding fruits like berries, oranges, or apples can also enhance flavor and nutrition.

- **Cook with seasonal produce:** Visit local farmers' markets to find seasonal fruits and vegetables. Incorporating seasonal produce into your meals supports local farmers and adds variety and flavor to your diet.

No Processed Foods

Processed foods often contain added sugars, unhealthy fats, and artificial ingredients that can lead to weight gain, insulin resistance, and other health issues. By avoiding these foods, residents maintain better metabolic health and lower their risk of developing chronic diseases such as heart disease, diabetes, and cancer.

Here are a few tips to help you avoid processed foods:

- **Shop the perimeter of the store:** Stick to the outer aisles where fresh produce, meats, dairy, and whole grains are typically located. The inner aisles often contain more processed and packaged foods.

- **Read labels carefully:** Take the time to read ingredient labels on packaged foods. A long list or having items that you cannot pronounce are signs that it is highly processed. Aim for products that have fewer ingredients, are recognizable, and are natural.

- **Prepare meals at home:** Cooking at home allows you to control the ingredients in your meals. Try simple recipes using fresh, whole foods. Meal prepping for the week can help you resist the temptation of convenience foods.

- **Snack smart:** Choose whole-food snacks instead of processed options. Keep healthy snacks such as fruits, yogurt, nuts, or cut vegetables available.

These tips can help you reduce your intake of processed foods and help you enhance your overall health.

Occasional Meat

Instead of being the main dish, meat is used sparingly, often in small portions to complement plant-based meals. This approach not only balances nutrient intake but also reduces the risk associated with high red and processed meat consumption, such as colorectal cancer and cardiovascular diseases.

People in Blue Zones typically opt for lean meats like poultry or fish rather than red meat. Follow these unique strategies to eat meat sparingly.

- **Use meat as a flavor enhancer:** Instead of being a centerpiece of a meal, use meat to add flavor. Add small amounts of bacon or lean sausage into soups, stews, or veggie dishes for added richness without relying on large portions.

- **Try meatless days:** Designate a few days a week to go meatless. This helps you explore new plant-based recipes, shifting your focus to grains, legumes, and vegetables while reserving meat for special occasions.

- **Stretch meat with plant-based ingredients:** Combine small portions of meat with larger amounts of beans, lentils, or mushrooms. These add bulk to dishes while keeping meat portions minimal.

- **Prioritize lean meats and fish:** Salmon or sardines are rich in omega-3 fatty acids, which support heart health and provide healthy fats. If you wish to include meat, opt for lean cuts such as chicken breast or turkey.

- **Use meat broth instead of meat chunks:** Add meat broth or stock into your cooking for flavor. This works well with soups, stews, and rice dishes, keeping meat portions minimal while still enjoying its taste.

Seafood and Water-Sourced Foods

Fish, particularly fatty fish such as salmon, mackerel, sardines, and tuna, are rich in omega-3 fatty acids. These healthy fats are crucial for brain health, reducing inflammation, and lowering the risk of heart disease. Studies have shown that regular seafood consumption can lead to improved cognitive function and decreased rates of depression, making it a vital part of the diet for aging populations (Leech, 2019).

Seaweed is another aquatic food embraced by several Blue Zone communities. A traditional staple in Okinawa, Japan, seaweed offers essential minerals such as iodine, iron, and calcium. Iodine is critical for thyroid function, which regulates metabolism and energy levels. Additionally, seaweed contains unique bioactive compounds that may help protect against certain cancers, improve gut health, and support cardiovascular health.

Water's Role in Diet and Practical Steps for Hydration

Our bodies rely on water for a multitude of vital functions, from aiding digestion to ensuring the efficient absorption of nutrients and facilitating toxin elimination. Without adequate hydration, these processes can falter, leading to a range of health issues.

Drink Only Quality Water Sources

Mineral-rich water and herbal teas are excellent choices as they provide more than just hydration; they offer additional health benefits. Mineral-rich water contains essential electrolytes like magnesium and calcium, which are crucial for muscle function, nerve transmission, and bone health.

Herbal teas, on the other hand, come with a variety of beneficial compounds depending on the herbs used. For example, chamomile tea can have calming effects and aid sleep, while peppermint tea can ease digestive discomfort.

- **Choose spring or filtered water:** Water from these sources has fewer impurities. Ensure that your water retains beneficial minerals such as calcium and magnesium.

- **Add natural mineral enhancers:** You can enhance the mineral content of filtered or distilled water by adding a few drops of trace mineral supplements. This boosts the electrolyte profile of water, supporting better hydration.

- **Drink water in a glass or stainless steel bottle:** Avoid plastic bottles that may leach harmful chemicals into your water. Instead, use glass or stainless steel containers to maintain the purity and quality of your water.

- **Monitor local water quality:** Stay informed about the water quality in your area by regularly checking reports. You may use a home water testing kit to detect any unwanted contaminants, ensuring your drinking water is safe and clean.

Avoid Sugary Drinks

Sugary beverages like sodas, energy drinks, and even some fruit juices are loaded with sugars and artificial ingredients that can lead to numerous health issues, including obesity and diabetes.

By choosing water or unsweetened herbal teas instead, you can avoid the empty calories and high sugar content that contribute to weight gain and blood sugar spikes. Moreover, water is calorie-free and promotes better hydration than sugary drinks, which can actually have a diuretic effect and contribute to dehydration. Follow these tips to make water more pleasant to drink.

- **Flavor water with fresh ingredients:** Add slices of fruit such as cucumber, lemon, or berries. You may also use herbs like mint or basil. This infuses water with natural flavors and encourages you to choose water instead of sugary beverages.

- **Dilute fruit juice:** If you crave fruit juice, dilute it with water to reduce the sugar content while still enjoying some of the flavor. A 50/50 mix cuts down sugar intake significantly while still offering a satisfying taste.

- **Carry a reusable water bottle:** Use an insulated, reusable water bottle that keeps water cold for hours. Having fresh water on hand helps you avoid sugary drinks when you're thirsty.

Eating Water-Rich Foods

Foods like cucumbers, melons, and seaweed have high water content and can complement your daily fluid intake. Cucumbers are composed of about 95% water and provide vitamins C and K as well as potassium and magnesium. Melons like watermelon and cantaloupe are similarly hydrating and contain antioxidants, vitamins, and minerals that support overall health.

- **Snack on water-rich veggies:** Keep cucumbers, celery, or bell peppers pre-sliced in the fridge for a quick, hydrating snack. Pair these with hummus or a yogurt dip for added flavor and nutrients.

- **Make hydrating salads:** Create salads with a base of water-dense greens such as iceberg or romaine lettuce, and top these with tomatoes, cucumbers, and radishes. Drizzle with a light vinaigrette for extra flavor.

- **Blend water-rich smoothies:** Add water-rich fruits such as watermelons, honeydew, or strawberries to your morning smoothie. These fruits boost hydration and provide natural sweetness without added sugars.

- **Include fruits as desserts:** Replace sugary desserts with a fresh bowl of fruit such as melons, grapes, or oranges. These fruits can satisfy your sweet cravings while adding vitamins and antioxidants to your diet.

- **Add seaweed into meals:** Add dried seaweed into soups, salads, or sushi rolls for a hydrating and nutrient-dense boost. Seaweed is packed with water, iodine, and minerals that support thyroid health and hydration.

Summary and Reflections

The diets of those in Blue Zones emphasize nutrient-dense whole foods such as whole grains, legumes, vegetables, fruits, seafood, and seaweed, which collectively support physical health and extend life expectancy.

Meanwhile, consuming mineral-rich water, herbal teas, and water-rich foods ensures the body receives essential nutrients while staying hydrated. By adopting these dietary and hydration practices, you can embrace a sustainable lifestyle that mirrors the habits of some of the world's longest-lived people, leading to improved quality of life and longevity.

Chapter 8:

Rest, Relaxation, and Blue Mindfulness

Rest, relaxation, and blue mindfulness are essential components of a balanced and healthy lifestyle. These practices help reduce stress and improve mental clarity and overall well-being. By understanding how to integrate these elements into daily life, you can create a routine that supports longevity and happiness.

Rest and Relaxation in Blue Zones

Daily naps are a common practice in many Blue Zones. In these areas, taking a nap is not seen as unproductive or lazy; rather, it is an essential part of the daily routine that contributes to overall well-being and longevity.

In Ikaria, Greece, napping is so ingrained in the culture that nearly everyone takes a midday siesta. Studies have shown that regular nappers have a lower risk of heart disease and other stress-related illnesses.

Naps Reset the Body

Naps provide a quick boost that can counteract the fatigue and stress accumulated during the day. A short nap of about 20 to 30 minutes can recharge your batteries without leaving you feeling groggy.

Regular relaxation practices also play an important role in reducing stress and lowering the risk of chronic diseases. Deep breathing exercises, meditation, and even simple moments of quiet reflection can activate the body's relaxation response, leading to lower blood pressure, reduced muscle tension, and improved mood.

A Relaxing Lifestyle

The people of Blue Zones have also cultivated lifestyles that naturally incorporate periods of rest and relaxation, rather than relegating them to specific times of the day. This seamless integration helps to maintain balanced cortisol levels throughout the day, which is crucial for managing stress and maintaining energy levels.

In Blue Zones, the culture often emphasizes the importance of pacing oneself and avoiding unnecessary stressors. This approach enables individuals to spend their energy judiciously, ensuring they remain sharp and focused when it matters most.

Daily Downtime

In Blue Zones, daily downtime is a key element of a long, healthy life. Taking intentional breaks from work and other stressors throughout the day allows the mind and body to reset.

Whether it's a few minutes of stepping outside for fresh air or simply sitting quietly with no distractions, these moments of unplugging can significantly reduce stress levels. This practice of regularly detaching from daily demands prevents burnout, promotes mental clarity, and encourages a deeper sense of peace, contributing to overall well-being.

Embracing Leisure

Leisure isn't a luxury in Blue Zones—it's a necessity. Engaging in enjoyable, low-stress activities such as gardening, walking, or spending time with loved ones is woven into the fabric of everyday life.

These moments of leisure offer more than just fun; they reduce the risk of heart disease, improve cognitive function, and promote emotional balance. By valuing leisure time, and avoiding the fast-paced, high-stress mentality found in other parts of the world, Blue Zone residents cultivate calmness and joy that supports longevity.

Mindful Moments

In Blue Zones, mindfulness and reflection play an essential role in promoting health and happiness. Practices like meditation, prayer, and moments of quiet contemplation help individuals manage stress and cultivate a positive outlook.

These mindful moments allow for introspection, emotional regulation, and mental restoration. By regularly engaging in these practices, Blue Zone residents maintain a strong connection to their inner peace, reducing the harmful effects of stress and contributing to both physical and emotional health.

Incorporating Blue Mind Practices Into Daily Life

Water has a natural ability to soothe the mind and body, thanks to its calming properties and the sensory experiences it provides.

Take Calming Baths

Immersing oneself in warm water has been shown to significantly reduce stress levels. The warmth helps to relax tense muscles, while the buoyancy can make you feel weightless, alleviating physical strain. Adding elements like essential oils, bath salts, or even soft lighting can enhance this experience, creating a sanctuary where worries can melt away.

Here are a few tips to enhance your bath experience, aligning it with Blue Mind principles.

- **Incorporate mindful breathing:** While in the bath, practice deep, mindful breathing. Focus on your breath, inhaling deeply through your nose and exhaling slowly. This will help you fully relax, calm your mind, and increase your awareness of the soothing water around you.

- **Use sounds of nature or soft music:** Play calming sounds of flowing water, ocean waves, or gentle rainfall in the background. These sounds can amplify the Blue Mind effect by engaging your auditory senses, making the experience even more tranquil.

- **Create a sensory ritual:** Enhance your bath with a sensory ritual by adding elements such as eucalyptus leaves, lavender essential oils, or candles with natural scents. These heighten the sensory connection to water, depending on relaxation and mental clarity.

Listen to Water

Whether it's the sound of ocean waves crashing on the shore, a gentle stream flowing through a forest, or rainfall on a rooftop, water sounds can transport you to a meditative state. These sounds have a rhythmic quality that mimics our body's natural rhythms, helping to slow down breathing and heart rates.

These techniques can help enhance your experience and deepen your connection to the Blue Mind principle.

- **Incorporate water sounds into your meditation practice:** Use water sounds as a background during meditation or mindfulness sessions. These gentle water rhythms can quiet your mind, allowing you to focus on your breathing and achieve a deeper state of relaxation.

- **Create a daily routine:** Set aside time each day to listen to water sounds. Whether during a work break or before bed. Regular exposure to these sounds can reduce stress, lower heart rate, and enhance mental clarity.

- **Pair water sounds with visualization:** Imagine yourself by the ocean or calm river to amplify the calming effects, making it easier to disconnect from stressors and tap into the restorative power of the Blue Mind concept.

Visit Local Bodies of Water

Taking a walk by a lake, river, or ocean can provide a peaceful environment perfect for reflection. The sight of glistening water and the sensation of a gentle breeze can work wonders for clearing the mind and grounding oneself. Consider these tips when visiting local bodies of water.

- **Engage your senses fully:** Feel the breeze on your skin, listen to the rhythmic sound of the water, and observe the movement of the waves or ripples. This helps you feel present and connected to nature, improving the water's calming effects.

- **Incorporate movement:** Activities such as walking, stretching, or yoga can reduce stress and boost mental and physical well-being.

- **Make it a routine:** Visit local bodies of water regularly, even for just a short time. Doing so can lower stress, improve mood, and align with the Blue Mind principles.

Concluding Thoughts

Integrating rest, relaxation, and water-based mindfulness into our daily routines can significantly enhance overall well-being. Regular rest periods, whether through short breaks or peaceful moments by local bodies of water, recharge our cognitive resources and foster a sense of contentment and purpose.

Embracing these habits not only supports overall health but also allows you to align with nature's rhythms, discovering a greater sense of peace and fulfillment in the process.

Chapter 9:

Creating Your Personal Blue Zone With Blue Mind Principles

Creating your personal Blue Zone with Blue Mind principles is about transforming your living space into a sanctuary for well-being. By making thoughtful choices in design and incorporating elements that promote tranquility, you can enhance both your mental and physical health.

Designing Your Environment

Bringing Blue Zone and Blue Mind elements into your surroundings can have a profound impact on your overall well-being.

Choose Calming Colors

Colors like blue and green can make your living space calm. These colors are known to promote tranquility and relaxation. Blue represents the sky and water, evoking a sense of calmness and peace. Green, on the other hand, symbolizes nature and renewal, making it an excellent choice for creating a serene environment.

- **Opt for soft, muted shades:** Go for pastel blues, sage greens, and light grays. These shades are less stimulating than bold or bright colors, helping you reduce stress and create a peaceful atmosphere. Soft blues mimic the open sky, while muted greens bring a subtle touch of nature indoors.

- **Use neutral bases with color accents:** Start with neutral colors such as soft beige, ivory, or pale gray for walls and large furniture pieces. Then, introduce calming colors like blue and green in accents such as cushions, artwork, and rugs. This allows you to maintain a peaceful base while adding touches of tranquility without overwhelming the space.

- **Consider earthy tones:** Colors such as light brown, sandy beige, and olive green can ground your environment in nature. These colors align with Blue Zone principles, promoting a sense of balance and connection to the earth. Earthy colors evoke feelings of warmth and stability, making your space feel more harmonious and calm.

Adding Natural Elements

Natural elements such as plants and water features can further enhance the calming effect of your space. Plants not only beautify your home but also improve air quality by filtering toxins and releasing oxygen. This can lead to better health and increased mental clarity.

Moreover, having plants indoors creates a connection with nature, which is essential for maintaining mental well-being. Simple additions like tabletop fountains or aquariums introduce the soothing sound of flowing water, which can be incredibly relaxing. Water features also add a dynamic element to the room, improving both its aesthetic appeal and ability to provide a calming sanctuary.

- **Choose low-maintenance plants:** Plants like snake plants, pothos, and peace lilies are easy to care for. These can thrive in various lighting conditions and require minimal attention. Adding low-maintenance plants ensures your space remains vibrant without adding stress, allowing you to enjoy their calming benefits without feeling overwhelmed by upkeep.

- **Create a green corner:** Design a specific area in your home as a "green corner" by grouping several plants together. Use varying heights and textures to create visual interest and depth. This can serve as your focal point, enhancing calmness, and providing a serene retreat for relaxation and reflection.

- **Incorporate water features:** Introduce tabletop fountains, wall-mounted water features, or aquariums to your space. The sound of flowing water has a natural soothing effect, reducing stress, and promoting tranquility, perfect for mindfulness and relaxation.

- **Use natural materials:** Add materials such as wood, stone, or bamboo to your decor and furniture choices. These materials connect your space to the outdoors and promote a sense of grounding and warmth. Natural textures also enhance a calm atmosphere, making your space more inviting and peaceful.

Having Ample Lighting

Natural light helps regulate your circadian rhythm, which in turn affects sleep patterns and overall mood. Exposure to sunlight boosts the production of serotonin, a hormone associated with happiness and well-being.

To optimize natural light, consider using sheer curtains that allow sunlight to filter through while still providing privacy. Positioning mirrors strategically can also help reflect light into darker corners of the room, enhancing the brightness and making the space feel more open and inviting. Here are more tips to improve lighting in your home.

- **Maximize window placement:** If you're designing a new space or renovating, prioritize large windows or skylights to bring in as much natural light as possible. Position windows strategically especially on south-facing walls (in the Northern Hemisphere) to ensure consistent sunlight throughout the day. This also improves mood and energy levels. Use glass doors to connect indoor and outdoor spaces for more natural light.

- **Utilize layered lighting:** Use ambient lighting (overhead fixtures), task lighting (lamps and reading lights), and accent lighting (decorative fixtures) to enhance overall illumination in the room. Layered lighting provides flexibility for different activities and maintains a cozy, tranquil environment during the evening.

- **Choose light-reflective surfaces:** Select light-colored walls, ceilings, and furniture to reflect natural light and brighten the space. Light tones such as whites, soft pastels, or light grays, amplify sunlight, making the area feel more open.

Additionally, incorporating reflective surfaces such as glass or polished metals can further enhance light distribution throughout the room.

Comfortable Furniture Arrangement

Start by assessing the layout of each room and identifying any obstacles that may hinder movement or make the space feel cluttered. Rearranging furniture to ensure easy flow and accessibility can make a significant difference.

Choose ergonomically designed furniture that supports good posture and reduces physical strain. Soft, cushioned seating options can make your living areas more inviting and conducive to relaxation. Creating designated zones for specific activities, such as reading, meditating, or socializing, can also help you utilize your space more efficiently.

- **Prioritize open spaces:** When arranging furniture, maintain clear pathways and open spaces for easy movement. Avoid placing large furniture pieces in high-traffic areas as this can create a sense of clutter and restrict flow. Aim for a layout that encourages movement, making the space feel more inviting and less chaotic. An open layout promotes calmness, allowing you to move through the room with ease.

- **Create intimate zones:** Designate specific areas within your room for different activities to enhance functionality and comfort. For example, arrange seating in a circular or semi-circular formation for social gatherings or a cozy nook with a chair and side table for reading and reflection.

- **Select comfortable seating options:** Choose furniture that supports good posture and promotes comfort. Sofas and chairs with ample cushioning encourage relaxation, while features such as lumbar support reduce physical strain during prolonged use. Doing so enhances the aesthetics of your space and invites you and your guests to relax and unwind.

Final Insights

Integrating Blue Zone and Blue Mind principles into your daily life can significantly enhance your well-being. By adopting calming colors, incorporating natural elements, ensuring ample natural light, and arranging comfortable, ergonomic furniture, you create a nurturing environment that promotes tranquility and relaxation.

These thoughtful design choices support emotional and physical health fostering a deeper connection with yourself and your surroundings.

Chapter 10:

Challenges and Solutions in Modern Life

Urban dwellers face various hurdles when trying to incorporate Blue Zone and Blue Mind practices into their lives. We will learn actionable strategies to integrate these wellness principles into even the most hectic schedules. Recognizing and addressing these challenges can help you find suitable approaches to enhance your well-being.

Obstacles to Blue Zone and Blue Mind Living

Urban living, characterized by crowded spaces and limited green areas, poses a significant challenge to incorporating Blue Zone and Blue Mind principles. Dense urban settings often restrict easy access to natural landscapes and bodies of water.

People residing in cities frequently find themselves surrounded by concrete jungles rather than serene parks or tranquil lakes. This scarcity of natural retreats discourages engagement in outdoor activities that foster physical well-being and mental relaxation.

Moreover, the hurried pace of city life is directly at odds with the slow, mindful approach championed by Blue Zone and Blue Mind lifestyles. Urban dwellers are often caught in a relentless cycle of work, commuting, and other responsibilities, leaving little time for leisure or reflective moments.

In addition to the physical constraints, modern conveniences like cars, computers, and smart gadgets contribute to increasingly sedentary habits. Transportation advancements have made walking or biking less common as people prefer the ease of driving or using public transit. Consequently, they miss out on the regular physical activity that is integral to maintaining health.

Overcoming Barriers Using Technology and Water Therapy

Incorporating Blue Zone and Blue Mind principles into modern life can seem daunting given the fast-paced and technology-driven nature of today's world. However, leveraging available technologies and adjusting our habits slightly can make these principles more accessible and practical.

Virtual Water Experience

For those who do not have regular access to natural bodies of water, virtual options like ocean videos or water-themed virtual reality (VR) can serve as substitutes. Research has shown that watching videos of water scenes—be it waves crashing on a beach or a tranquil river flowing through a forest—can significantly reduce stress and lower heart rates (Jo, 2019).

Consider these strategies to create your own virtual water experience.

- **Create a virtual retreat space:** Designate a specific area in your home for virtual water experiences. You can use a comfortable chair, soft lighting, and calming decor. Set up a screen or projector to display ocean videos or calming water scenes, creating an immersive environment that encourages relaxation.

- **Utilize water sounds in daily life:** Incorporate the soothing sounds of water into your everyday routine. Use apps or online resources to play ambient sounds of ocean waves, babbling brooks, or rain while working, meditating, or relaxing. These calming auditory elements mimic the experience of being near water, promoting stress relief and enhancing your mood even in non-water settings.

- **Engage with water-themed activities:** These can be activities such as painting or drawing water scenes, engaging in mindfulness exercises that visualize being near water, or practicing yoga poses that mimic the fluidity of water movement. By immersing in these activities, you create a connection to the calming aspects of water, enhancing your overall well-being.

Water Visualization

Incorporating micro-breaks with water visualization can play a crucial role in reducing stress and enhancing mental clarity. Taking short breaks throughout the day to close one's eyes and imagine being near water, or listening to recordings of water sounds like rain or a babbling brook, can offer significant psychological benefits.

- **Schedule regular micro-breaks:** Set aside times throughout the day for short micro-breaks dedicated to water visualization. Even just five minutes can be effective. Use a timer to remind yourself to step away from work or daily tasks. During these breaks, close your eyes, take a few deep breaths, and visualize yourself near a peaceful body of water.

- **Create a calming environment:** Find a quiet and comfortable spot where you can relax without distractions. Consider dimming the lights, using a comfortable chair or cushion, and adding elements that evoke water themes such as pictures of serene lakes or ocean scenes.

- **Combine visualization with breathing techniques:** As you visualize a calming water scene, synchronize your breath with the imagery—inhale deeply as you imagine waves gently rolling in, and exhale as you envision them retreating. This visualization and breathing technique enhances relaxation and clears your mind, improving mental clarity.

Using Technology and Apps

Apps like Calm and Headspace include sections dedicated to water sounds, such as waves, waterfalls, and rainfall. These sounds are proven to have calming effects, aiding in meditation practices and bedtime routines.

More advanced gadgets, such as ambient sound machines or sleep therapy systems, create personalized environments conducive to relaxation by combining water sounds with other calming elements like soft lighting. Consider these techniques when using technology and apps to promote Blue Zone and Blue Mind principles.

- **Choose the right app for your needs:** Explore meditation and relaxation apps that offer dedicated sections for water sounds. Whether you want to enhance focus during the day or unwind before bed, these apps allow you to customize your experience with specific water themes such as ocean waves, rivers, or rain. Experiment with different sounds and settings to find the ones that resonate most with you, helping you integrate Blue Mind practices seamlessly into your daily life.

- **Set up sleep therapy and water sounds:** Utilize advanced gadgets such as sound machines or sleep therapy systems to create a relaxing sleep movement. Many of these devices offer water-themed soundscapes paired with soft, adjustable lighting. Set the device to play gentle rain or waves before bedtime to help you fall asleep faster and enjoy a deeper rest. Sound machines can also be programmed to gradually reduce volume as you drift off, ensuring an uninterrupted peaceful sleep experience.

- **Create a personalized relaxation routine:** Use technology to create a customized relaxation routine that fits your lifestyle. Combine water sounds, soft lighting, and breathing exercises in apps or sound machines to create a holistic experience. Set timers for short breaks during the day to use water sounds for stress relief, or program your device for longer evening sessions to unwind and relax before bed.

Holistic health tracking devices that monitor stress levels and recommend breaks based on one's physiological data can be particularly useful for maintaining a balanced lifestyle.

Water Therapy

Water therapy can be an effective solution for overcoming barriers to implementing Blue Zone and Blue Mind principles, especially for individuals with limited access to natural bodies of water. Incorporating water into daily routines can provide the calming and restorative benefits associated with Blue Mind practices.

These activities reduce stress, promote mental clarity, and encourage a connection to nature, even in urban environments.

- **Incorporate regular baths or showers:** Turn daily baths or showers into a mindful experience. Focus on the sensation of water on your skin and its calming effects. Adding essential oils or bath salts can enhance relaxation, creating a water therapy session that reduces stress and refreshes your mind and body.

- **Engage in water-based exercises:** If you have access to a pool, incorporate water-based exercises such as swimming or water aerobics into your fitness routine. These activities are gentle on the joints and provide both physical and mental health benefits, promoting relaxation while keeping you active.

- **Try hydrotherapy techniques:** Use simple hydrotherapy techniques such as alternating warm and cold water in the shower to improve circulation and reduce muscle tension. This technique is known to relieve stress and promote relaxation, allowing you to enjoy water therapy without needing special equipment.

- **Create a virtual water experience:** If you cannot access water regularly, stimulate the calming effects through technology. Play water sounds or watch videos of tranquil rivers or oceans during breaks or relaxation periods. This virtual experience can help replicate the stress-relieving benefits of natural water settings, supporting mental well-being.

By making water therapy accessible, individuals can experience the health and well-being advantages of Blue Zone living no matter their location.

Final Thoughts

Urban living and the fast-paced demands of modern life present significant challenges to adopting Blue Zone and Blue Mind principles. Adopting practical solutions can make these principles more accessible. By adapting these strategies to fit personal lifestyles, achieving a balance of longevity and well-being becomes more attainable in a modern environment.

Chapter 11:

The Future of Blue Living

Let's explore various strategies for creating urban landscapes that align with Blue Zone and Blue Mind principles. In this chapter, we will highlight green infrastructure and how these can serve as communal hubs for physical activities and social interaction. We will also learn how incorporating water into urban environments can shape the future of public health and urban living.

My Family's Legacy on Lake Champlain

In 1953, when the U.S. government decommissioned the lighthouse station on Juniper Island in Lake Champlain, my father seized the chance to preserve a piece of history. He submitted the winning bid at the auction and, by 1956, became the proud owner of the 12-acre island, just 3 ½ miles west of Burlington's waterfront.

Juniper Island became more than a family treasure—it symbolized our connection to the lake and the importance of safeguarding water spaces for future generations. It's a reminder that preserving these natural sanctuaries promotes the peace, clarity, and "Blue Mind" that only water can provide.

Potential for Urban Blue Zones

Urban environments that foster Blue Zone and Blue Mind principles can significantly enhance the quality of life by promoting relaxation, physical health, and community well-being.

Adding Natural Water Sources to Cityscapes

Rivers, lakes, and even man-made ponds and fountains can create serene spaces where people can unwind and find mental peace. For example, the Riverwalk in San Antonio, Texas, seamlessly blends the urban environment with the natural beauty of a winding river, offering locals and tourists alike an oasis in the heart of the city.

Here are more ideas to add natural water sources to structures in your city or community.

- **Green roof ponds and water gardens:** Integrating rooftop water features such as small ponds or water gardens into roofs can transform unused urban spaces into tranquil natural areas. These water elements enhance the aesthetic value and contribute to biodiversity by attracting birds and insects while aiding in temperature regulation and reducing urban heat islands.

- **Restorative urban wetlands:** Reviving or creating small wetlands in underutilized urban spaces, such as vacant lots or parks, can provide natural filtration systems for stormwater while offering habitats for wildlife. These wetlands act as peaceful retreats where city dwellers can reconnect with nature, fostering relaxation and mental clarity.

- **Floating parks on waterways:** Cities with rivers, lakes, or coastal access can develop floating parks that merge water with greenery. These innovative parks provide recreational space for walking, meditation, or yoga, while also highlighting the water's natural beauty. Floating parks such as Rotterdam's Floating Forest exemplify how urban water sources can become lively public spaces.

- **Waterfront redevelopment with public access:** Transforming industrial or neglected waterfronts into public spaces with boardwalks, piers, or terraced seating along rivers and lakes can enhance landscapes. By improving access to natural water bodies, these areas can be revitalized for community gatherings, outdoor dining, or leisure activities.

- **Urban canals with integrated public spaces:** Cities can design new or renovate existing canals that flow through neighborhoods and business districts, creating linear parks along the water. Incorporating walking paths, cafes, and outdoor seating alongside the canals, like Amsterdam's network of waterways, encourages physical activity, relaxation, and social interaction with water as a central, calming feature.

Green Infrastructure

Parks serve as communal grounds where people can engage in physical activities like jogging, cycling, or yoga, thus promoting physical health. Central Park in New York City is a prime example of how large green spaces can provide recreational opportunities and vital connections among urban dwellers. Here are green infrastructure ideas you can apply to your city or community.

- **Multi-functional green corridors:** Transform unused urban land, such as old rail lines or utility corridors, into green pathways that connect different parts of the city. This promotes physical activity and serves as nature-filled commutes. Green corridors can include walking, jogging, and cycling paths, as well as outdoor gyms, public art, and community gardens, fostering social connections while offering easy access to recreational spaces. The High Line in NYC is a successful example of this concept, blending green infrastructure with urban convenience.

- **Urban agricultural parks:** Converting vacant lots or underutilized spaces into community farming parks enables residents to grow their food while encouraging physical activity. These parks can host raised vegetable beds, fruit trees, and herbs, alongside areas for yoga and outdoor exercise classes. By combining green space with local food production, urban agriculture parks improve access to healthy food, enhance sustainability, and create gathering spots for the community.

- **Vertical green spaces on building facades:** Incorporating vertical gardens or living walls into building facades offers a creative solution for adding green space in highly dense urban areas with limited horizontal space. These vertical green spaces beautify the environment, improve air quality, reduce noise pollution, and encourage physical interaction with nature. Residents or office workers nearby can benefit from the calming effects of greenery even in a compact urban environment.

- **Pop-up green spaces:** Introducing temporary, mobile green spaces, such as "pop-up parks" or "parklets," can revitalize urban areas that lack permanent green infrastructure. These mobile green spaces can include small grass lawns, potted plants, seating areas, and shade trees. They provide instant access to nature for pedestrians, cyclists, and local residents, encouraging outdoor activities such as yoga, picnics, or relaxation while bringing greenery to previously concrete-heavy zones.

Sustainable Architectural Practices

Buildings that integrate aquatic elements like indoor waterfalls, rooftop gardens with water features, or rainwater harvesting systems create visually appealing spaces and encourage mindfulness and environmental responsibility. The Bosco Verticale in Milan, Italy, exemplifies how innovative design and sustainable practices can coexist; its towers are home to thousands of plants and trees, creating a vertical forest that improves air quality and provides visually stimulating environments for residents. Let us explore these ideas in the following sustainable architectural strategies.

- **Rainwater harvesting and irrigation system:** Designing buildings with integrated rainwater harvesting systems can capture and store rainwater for reuse in irrigation, plumbing, and rooftop water features. Collected rainwater can be used to maintain rooftop gardens, vertical green walls, or indoor water elements, promoting sustainability while reducing reliance on municipal water supplies.

- **Indoor waterfalls and green atriums:** Incorporating indoor waterfalls or water features within building atriums adds visual appeal and also promotes a calming, nature-infused atmosphere. These features can enhance air humidity and create tranquil spaces for mindfulness and relaxation. Pairing water elements with natural light and indoor plant installations, such as living walls, creates biophilic spaces that reconnect occupants with nature.

- **Rooftop wetlands for filtration:** Utilizing rooftop space for constructed wetlands or bioswales is a sustainable way to filter greywater from the building's systems. These wetlands act as natural filters for water before it's reused for irrigation or safely released back into the environment. By combining wetland plants with rooftop water features, the building can integrate aquatic biodiversity, enhancing the aesthetic value of the space while reducing water waste.

Blue Mind and Public Health Advocacy

Advocating for water accessibility and protection of aquatic environments is essential to achieve the broader goals within Blue Zones and Blue Mind principles. To build a future where urban living supports public health, begin with policies that ensure everyone has access to clean and safe water.

Create Equitable Access

Equitable access means that no community, regardless of socioeconomic status, should be without this fundamental resource. Implementing these policies might involve local governments prioritizing infrastructure projects aimed at upgrading aging water supply systems or introducing new technologies to purify water. Here are techniques to apply equitable access to clean and safe water.

- **Sliding scale water pricing models:** Implementing a sliding scale for water pricing, based on income levels, ensures that all households can afford clean water regardless of their financial situation. This helps subsidize the cost of water for low-income communities while maintaining fair pricing for those who can afford higher rates. This system allows equitable water access while generating revenue for necessary infrastructure improvements.

- **Community-owned water cooperatives:** Establishing community-owned water cooperatives in underserved areas empowers residents to manage and maintain their water resources. These cooperatives can be funded by local governments or non-profit organizations, with the community playing a central role in decision-making. This model encourages sustainable water management practices, promotes local accountability, and ensures that water remains a public resource rather than being privatized.

- **Mobile water purification stations:** Deploying mobile water purification stations to areas with limited access to clean water can offer immediate relief while longer-term infrastructure projects are underway. These portable stations can purify water from local sources or rainwater and distribute it to residents. By bringing clean water directly to those in need, this addresses the gap in access in remote or impoverished communities.

Supporting Conservation Efforts

Healthy water bodies are indispensable for both ecological balance and human well-being. Organizations dedicated to conservation work tirelessly to safeguard endangered species, restore degraded habitats, and combat pollution. Policy-makers and community leaders can reinforce these objectives by enacting regulations that minimize industrial discharge into rivers and lakes, thus promoting sustainable agricultural practices that prevent nutrient runoff. Consider these strategies:

- **Incentivizing sustainable agricultural practices:** Governments can introduce financial incentives, such as tax breaks or subsidies, for farmers who adopt sustainable practices that minimize nutrient runoff into water bodies. Techniques such as over-cropping, reduced use of chemical fertilizers, and buffer zones with native vegetation help reduce pollutants entering rivers and lakes. By rewarding eco-friendly farming practices, this strategy helps protect aquatic ecosystems and promotes long-term conservation efforts.

- **Implementing strict industrial discharge regulations:** Enforcing strict regulations on industrial discharge and requiring companies to treat wastewater before releasing it into natural water bodies can drastically reduce pollution levels. Regular monitoring and penalties for non-compliance ensure accountability. Additionally, encouraging industries to adopt closed-loop water systems, where water is reused within the production process, further reduces environmental impacts.

- **Public-private partnerships for wetland and watershed restoration:** Collaborating with private companies and non-profit organizations, governments can support large-scale wetland and watershed restoration projects. Wetlands naturally filter pollutants, provide habitat for wildlife, and prevent flooding. Public-private partnerships can fund and implement the restoration of degraded areas, combining resources and expertise to strengthen conservation efforts and restore ecological balance in affected regions.

Community Participation

People can engage in various activities such as volunteer clean-up drives, citizen science projects monitoring water quality, or advocacy groups lobbying for stricter environmental protections.

Schools and local organizations can lead workshops educating citizens on the simple ways they can make a difference. When individuals understand the impact of their actions, they become powerful advocates for change within their own neighborhoods. Here are more ideas.

- **Neighborhood clean-up events with educational components:** Organize regular community clean-up drives focused on local rivers, lakes, or coastal areas. These events can include short educational sessions on the importance of keeping water bodies clean and how litter impacts aquatic systems. By combining hands-on involvement with learning, participants are more likely to internalize the value of their efforts and spread awareness to others.

- **Citizen science water monitoring programs:** Encourage citizens to participate in water quality monitoring projects where they can collect and submit data on local water bodies. These projects can track pollutants, temperature changes, and wildlife health, providing valuable information to environmental scientists. Equipping residents with simple testing kits and online platforms for data entry fosters direct involvement in conservation while empowering communities to monitor the health of their local environment.

- **Local water conservation workshops:** Schools, community centers, and local organizations can offer workshops on water conservation techniques, teaching residents how to reduce water waste in their daily lives. Topics like installing low-flow fixtures, using rain barrels, or creating xeriscape gardens that require less water can be covered. These workshops provide practical tools for individuals to make a measurable difference at home, while also promoting collective responsibility for sustainable water use.

- **Youth-led environmental advocacy groups:** Forming youth-led environmental clubs within schools or community groups can create a new generation of advocates for clean water. These groups can lobby local governments for stricter environmental protections, organize awareness campaigns, or collaborate with other local organizations for water-related causes. Youth involvement ensures long-term sustainability and fosters a culture of activism that encourages peers and community members to engage in water conservation efforts.

Enhancing Mental and Physical Health

Activities like swimming, kayaking, or even leisurely walks by a pond can greatly contribute to one's well-being. Communities that prioritize the creation and maintenance of such recreational opportunities enable their residents to reap the benefits of regular connection with aquatic environments.

Communities must create symbiotic relationships between land and water-based wellness initiatives, thus creating a seamless blend of healthy living practices.

Medical Breakthroughs

The goal of this book is to explore how our interaction with water, through the principles of Blue Zone and Blue Mind practices, can enhance physical and emotional well-being while contributing to increased human longevity.

Alongside these natural practices, it's important to consider emerging scientific research, such as the drug Rapamycin, which holds the potential to complement these principles. By promoting cognitive health, cardiovascular function, and reducing age-related decline, Rapamycin could serve as a modern tool that supports the natural, holistic approaches found in Blue Zone lifestyles.

Rapamycin Overview

Rapamycin was originally used as an immunosuppressant to prevent organ rejection. It has recently garnered attention for its potential to extend lifespan and improve age-related health outcomes, aligning with Blue Zone values of longevity and well-being.

Key Findings on Rapamycin's Impact on Longevity

- **Mechanism of action:** Rapamycin inhibits the mTOR pathway, a regulator of cell growth and aging, and has been shown to extend lifespan in organisms like mice, fruit flies, and worms.

- **Preclinical animal studies:** In mice and other animals, Rapamycin improves healthspan markers such as cardiovascular function and cognitive performance, mirroring the benefits of Blue Zone practices.

- **Human trials:** Early human trials are exploring the safety, dosage, and efficacy of Rapamycin, with some evidence suggesting it can enhance immune function in older adults.

- **Effects on age-related diseases:** Rapamycin may help prevent cognitive decline, improve cardiovascular health, and reduce skin aging, addressing key aspects of aging seen in Blue Zone populations.

Side Effects and Future Directions

Despite its promise, Rapamycin's side effects such as immunosuppression and metabolic concerns, must be carefully managed. Future research focuses on optimizing strategies, developing safer rapalogs, and combining Rapamycin with other therapies to promote longevity.

Rapalogs are a class of drugs that mimic the effects of rapamycin. These drugs are designed to target similar pathways as rapamycin but with potentially fewer side effects, making them promising in anti-aging and therapeutic research.

Final Thoughts

Rapamycin could potentially bridge the gap between modern science and natural practices. While animal studies strongly support its role in lifespan extension, human studies are just beginning. Combining Rapamycin with Blue Zone and Blue Mind principles could provide a balanced approach to achieving longer, healthier lives.

Bringing It All Together

Integrating Blue Zones and Blue Mind principles into urban living by weaving natural water sources like rivers, lakes, and ponds into cityscapes, can nurture relaxation, physical health, and community cohesion.

Everyone must advocate for water accessibility and protect aquatic ecosystems to support public health. Policies ensuring equitable access to clean water and public awareness campaigns about the mental health benefits of being near water are crucial steps.

Community participation can help safeguard these resources. Together, these strategies exemplify how cities can create resilient systems that prioritize the well-being of their residents through thoughtful integration of water and nature.

Conclusion

As we draw to the end of this exploration of *The Blue Connection*—the remarkable influence of water on longevity, well-being, and overall quality of life—let's turn our attention to the future.

How do we take these insights and translate them into actionable steps that can transform our daily lives and communities?

Let's Create Blue Zones in Our Communities

Imagine bustling urban centers transformed by principles inspired by the world's Blue Zones, areas where people live significantly longer and healthier lives. Picture cities with easily accessible green spaces interspersed with serene water features such as fountains, ponds, and riverside trails.

These environments encourage physical activity and provide mental reprieve from the stresses of urban living

- Urban policies could prioritize the conversion of underused areas into community gardens with small water elements or renovate parks to include natural swimming ponds.

- Schools, workplaces, and residential buildings could also embrace Blue Zone ideas by incorporating spaces designed with water features, like meditation gardens with flowing streams or rooftop pools.

- Investing in water-focused public art, such as interactive fountains or rain gardens, can also create communal focal points, bringing people together and strengthening community bonds.

These environments enhance aesthetic appeal and imbue daily routines with moments of tranquility and mindfulness, fostering both mental and physical health.

Improve Health and Wellness With Blue Mind Wisdom

Water-related activities can help reduce stress and improve mental well-being. Public health campaigns should actively champion access to clean, safe water for recreational purposes, promoting these activities as not just leisurely pursuits but integral components of healthy living.

Local governments and healthcare providers can collaborate to organize community events centered around water, including beach clean-ups, group swims, or kayaking excursions, thereby promoting an active lifestyle while fostering a sense of community stewardship for natural water resources.

Promote Access to Clean Drinking Water

Advocating for improved water infrastructure in underserved areas helps address significant health disparities and underscores the intrinsic link between water accessibility and community wellness. Policies supporting water conservation and the protection of aquatic ecosystems ensure that current and future generations can continue to benefit from the rejuvenating properties of natural water bodies.

Support Initiatives to Protect Bodies of Water

Supporting organizations and initiatives that aim to protect bodies of water—from local lakes and rivers to oceans—safeguards these vital resources against pollution and depletion. It's a rallying cry for joining forces with environmental groups, participating in local water conservancy projects, and lobbying for stricter regulations on industrial pollutants and waste management.

Considering Medical Breakthroughs

Rapamycin offers an exciting scientific complement to the natural, holistic principles of Blue Zone and Blue Mind principles, potentially enhancing human longevity by providing cognitive health, and cardiovascular function, and reducing age-related decline in animal studies. The drug is beginning to show promise in human trials, particularly in supporting immune function and preventing age-related diseases.

However, its side effects such as immunosuppression, highlight the need for careful dosage management and further research. Combining Rapamycin's modern breakthroughs with the time-tested practices of water-based well-being could provide a powerful, balanced approach to living longer, healthier lives.

Creating Spaces and Lifestyles That Honor the Importance of Water

The knowledge gleaned from Blue Zones and Blue Mind principles calls for an unwavering commitment to integrating water into the fabric of our everyday existence, fostering environments that nurture longevity and holistic well-being.

We need active participation and dedication from everyone. Start small—introduce houseplants that thrive in water, install a water feature in your garden, or carve out time for regular visits to local waterfronts. Teach children the value of water through interactive lessons and family outings to natural aquatic spots, fostering the next generation's appreciation for these invaluable resources.

Communities can begin organizing events aimed at raising awareness about the significance of water in promoting health and happiness. Form neighborhood walking groups that explore nearby water bodies, create social media campaigns encouraging water-centric lifestyle changes, or host educational workshops offering practical advice on incorporating water's benefits into daily routines.

The Power of Water Is Within Us

The power of water in fostering long, healthy lives and enriching our well-being is undeniable. By embracing the insights from Blue Zones and Blue Mind science, we can reshape our environments and habits profoundly.

It requires vision, collaborative spirit, and sustained effort, but the rewards—a healthier, more connected, and vibrant existence—are well worth it.

The journey towards a future where water plays a central role in enhancing the quality of life begins now, with each one of us taking deliberate steps to weave the essence of Blue Living into the fabric of our communities and personal lifestyles.

Let us move forward in creating a world where the transformative power of water is harnessed for the benefit of all.

References

Berman, R. (2022, November 21). *Having a sense of purpose may help you live longer, research shows.* Medical News Today. https://www.medicalnewstoday.com/articles/longevity-having-a-purpose-may-help-you-live-longer-healthier

Bishop, R. (2023, March 15). *Does purpose play a positive role in mental health?* Mayo Clinic Health System. Retrieved October 15, 2024, from https://www.mayoclinichealthsystem.org/hometown-health/speaking-of-health/purpose-and-mental-health

Blue zones project challenges. (n.d.). Blue Zones Project. https://lakecounty.bluezonesproject.com/challenges/

Brainz Magazine. (2022, March 17). *Creating your own blue zone.* Brainz Magazine. www.brainzmagazine.com/post/creating-your-own-blue-zone

Caruso, C. Ligotti, M. E., Accardi, G., Aiello, A., Duro, G., Galimberti, D., & Candore, G. (2022). How important are genes to achieve longevity? *International Journal of Molecular Sciences, 23*(10), 5635. https://doi.org/10.3390/ijms23105635

Chan, A. (2019, December 3). *Creating community: The role of green and blue spaces in cities.* Yale Environment Review. https://environment-review.yale.edu/creating-community-role-green-and-blue-spaces-cities

Diamond, J. (2023, October 16). *Adopting a blue zones way of life: What you need to do to survive the challenges we face today.* MenAlive. https://menalive.com/adopting-a-blue-zones-way-of-life/

Dive into health: Exploring the benefits of water activities. (2024, May 2). My Boat Life. www.myboatlife.com/2024/05/dive-into-health-exploring-the-benefits-of-water-activities.html

Fields, H. (2011, October 31). *Happiness associated with longer life.* Science. www.science.org/content/article/happiness-associated-longer-life.

Haeffner, M., Jackson-Smith, D., Buchert, M., & Risley, J. (2017). Accessing blue spaces: Social and geographic factors structuring familiarity with, use of, and appreciation of urban waterways. *Landscape and Urban Planning, 167*, 136–146. https://doi.org/10.1016/j.landurbplan.2017.06.008

Hindle, G., & Hindle, G. (2019, May 17). *What is cannonau? Ask Decanter.* Decanter. https://www.decanter.com/learn/advice/what-is-cannonau-413919/

History of blue zones. (n.d.). Blue Zones. https://www.bluezones.com/about/history/

Hydrotherapy and mental health: Therapeutic benefits of water. (2024, August 16). HydroWorx. www.hydroworx.com/blog/hydrotherapy-and-mental-health-the-therapeutic-benefits-of-water/

Imatome-Yun, N. (2024, August 2). *Hara hachi bu: Enjoy food and lose weight with this simple Japanese phrase.* Blue Zones. https://www.bluezones.com/2017/12/hara-hachi-bu-enjoy-food-and-lose-weight-with-this-simple-phrase/

Jo, H., Song, C., & Miyazaki, Y. (2019). Physiological Benefits of Viewing Nature: A Systematic review of indoor experiments. *International Journal of Environmental Research and Public Health*, *16*(23), 4739. https://doi.org/10.3390/ijerph16234739

Keogh, B. (n.d.). *Secrets of longevity from the blue zones.* Mindful Living With Bernadette. https://mindfulliving.coach/secrets-of-longevity-from-the-blue-zones/

Kotifani, A. (2018, December 11). *The future of urban living: Building and shaping great cities.* Blue Zones. www.bluezones.com/2018/12/the-future-of-urban-living-building-and-shaping-great-cities/.

Kotifani, A. (2022, September 26). *Moai—This tradition is why Okinawan people live longer, better.* Blue Zones. https://www.bluezones.com/2018/08/moai-

this-tradition-is-why-okinawan-people-live-
longer-better/

Latham, F. (2022, November 10). *The surprising benefits of blue spaces.* BBC. https://www.bbc.com/future/article/20221108 -the-doctors-prescribing-blue-therapy

Leech, J. (2019, June 11). *11 evidence-based health benefits of eating fish.* Healthline. https://www.healthline.com/nutrition/11- health-benefits-of-fish#TOC_TITLE_HDR_2

Leech, J. (2020, June 30). *7 science-based health benefits of drinking enough water.* Healthline. www.healthline.com/nutrition/7-health- benefits-of-water.

Lovato, N., & Lack, L. (2010). The effects of napping on cognitive functioning. *Progress in Brain Research,* 155–166. https://doi.org/10.1016/b978-0-444- 53702-7.00009-9

McIntosh, J. (2018, July 16). *15 benefits of drinking water and other water facts.* Medical News Today. www.medicalnewstoday.com/articles/290814.

Mikstas, C. (2023, February 3). *Seven wonders of water.* WebMD. https://www.webmd.com/diet/ss/slideshow- water-health

Moday Center. (2019, January 29) *Design your health: Create your own blue zone.*

modaycenter.com/2019/01/29/design-your-health-create-your-own-blue-zone/

Nichols, J., W. (2014). *Blue Mind.* Little, Brown and Company.

Our guide to creating your own blue zone. (2024, August 30). The Terraces at Bonita Springs. www.theterracesatbonitasprings.com/2024/08/30/guide-to-creating-your-own-blue-zone/

Popkin, B. M., D'Anci, K. E., & Rosenberg, I. H. (2010). Water, hydration, and health. *Nutrition Reviews, 68*(8), 439–458. https://doi.org/10.1111/j.1753-4887.2010.00304.x

Robertson, R. (2017, August 29) *Why people in "blue zones" live longer than the rest of the world.* Healthline. www.healthline.com/nutrition/blue-zones

Rosinger, A. Y. (2021). The human thirst. *Scientific American, 325*(1), 38. https://doi.org/10.1038/scientificamerican0721-38

Self-guided relaxation exercises for anxiety, depression and wellbeing management. (n.d.). Beyond Blue. https://www.beyondblue.org.au/mental-health/wellbeing/relaxation-exercises

Simon-Thomas, E. (2015, December 18). *Does happiness really help you live longer?* Greater Good Magazine. https://greatergood.berkeley.edu/article/item/does_happiness_really_help_you_live_longer

Song, C. F., Tay, P. K. C., Gwee, X., Wee, S. L., & Ng, T. P. (2023). Happy people live longer because they are healthy people. *BMC Geriatrics, 23*(1). https://doi.org/10.1186/s12877-023-04030-w

Song, I., Baek, K., Kim, C., & Song, C. (2023). Effects of nature sounds on the attention and physiological and psychological relaxation. *Urban Forestry & Urban Greening, 86,* 127987. https://doi.org/10.1016/j.ufug.2023.127987

Unlocking the secrets of blue zones: A blueprint for longevity and health. (2023, September 20). News-Medical. www.news-medical.net/health/Unlocking-the-Secrets-of-Blue-Zones-A-Blueprint-for-Longevity-and-Health.aspx.

Vieira, N. M., Peghinelli, V. V., Monte, M. G., Costa, N. A., Pereira, A. G., Seki, M. M., Azevedo, P. S., Polegato, B. F., De Paiva, S. a. R., Zornoff, L. a. M., & Minicucci, M. F. (2023). Beans comsumption can contribute to the prevention of cardiovascular disease. *Clinical Nutrition ESPEN, 54,* 73–80. https://doi.org/10.1016/j.clnesp.2023.01.007

What are blue zones? (n.d.). Max Planck Institute for Biology of Ageing. https://www.age.mpg.de/what-are-blue-zones

What is Pecorino cheese? What does Pecorino taste like? (n.d.). Cheese.com. https://www.cheese.com/pecorino/

Zhang, X., Zhang, Y., Zhai, J., Wu, Y., & Mao, A. (2021). Waterscapes for promoting mental health in the general population. *International Journal of Environmental Research and Public Health*, *18*(22), 11792. https://doi.org/10.3390/ijerph182211792

www.ingramcontent.com/pod-product-compliance
Lightning Source LLC
Chambersburg PA
CBHW060922140726
47996CB00001B/337